Trusted advice

Preparing **for childbirth**

A practical guide to childbirth choices

DRmiriam**stoppard**

LONDON, NEW YORK, MUNICH,
MELBOURNE, AND DELHI

Author's dedication: For Kate

Revised Edition
Assistant Editor Dharini
Editors Bushra Ahmed, Sreshtha Bhattacharya
Assistant Designer Arijit Ganguly
Designer Anchal Kaushal
Senior Designers Tannishtha Chakraborty,
Sudakshina Basu
Managing Editor Suchismita Banerjee
Design Manager Arunesh Talapatra
DTP Operator Vishal Bhatia
DTP Designers Pushpak Tyagi, Nand Kishor Acharya,
Mohammad Usman
DTP Manager Sunil Sharma
Picture Researcher Sakshi Saluja

Project Editor Daniel Mills
Senior Art Editors Isabel de Cordova, Edward Kinsey
Managing Editor Penny Warren
Managing Art Editor Glenda Fisher
Publisher Peggy Vance
Senior Production Editor Jennifer Murray
Creative Technical Support Sonia Charbonnier
Senior Production Controller Man Fai Lau

First published by Dorling Kindersley in 1998
Reprinted 2001

This revised edition published in Great Britain in 2012
by Dorling Kindersley Limited
80 Strand, London WC2R ORL A Penguin Company

001–178123–02/2012

A CIP catalogue record for this book is available
from the British Library.

ISBN 978-1-4053-5647-3

Reproduced by Colourscan, Singapore
Printed in China by Leo Paper

Discover more at
www.dk.com

Contents

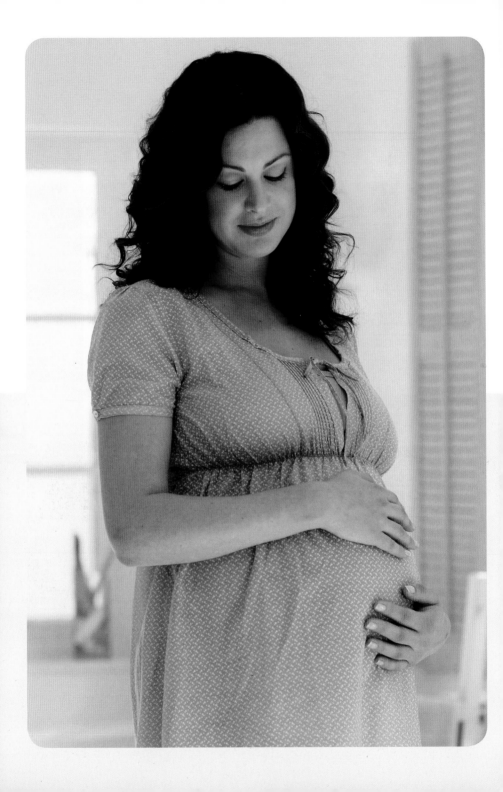

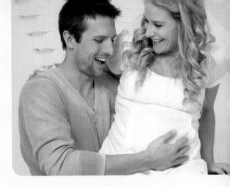

Chapter 4

Your baby is born 51

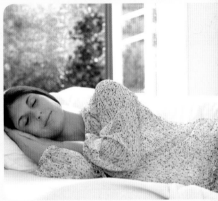

Chapter 5

Special circumstances 63

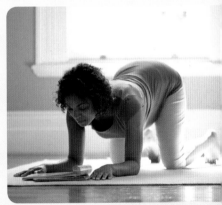

Chapter 6

Getting back to normal 81

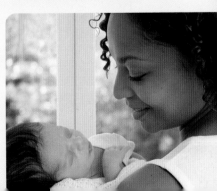

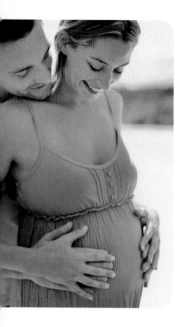

Introduction

Giving birth to your baby is an exciting and emotional event, but even if it isn't your first time, you'll probably approach the actual birth with some trepidation. Will I know when I'm in labour? Will it be very painful? How long will it take? There are so many questions to be answered and decisions to be made, and with the help of this book you'll have straightforward and constructive advice to help you through this momentous event.

In theory it's possible to have exactly the kind of birth that you want. Most women give birth in hospital, where medical back-up is readily available, but nowadays a hospital birth needn't be a high-tech impersonal affair. Giving birth at home is once again becoming more widely accepted, especially with the increasing use of locally based community midwife care. Think about how you want your birth to be and draw up a birth plan outlining your preferences in consultation with your caregivers, but remember to be flexible.

Preparation

Prepare for the birth by attending your regular antenatal appointments and joining classes run either at your hospital clinic, or by independent midwives or childbirth experts. These give you invaluable information about labour and birth, and how your birth partner can help support you throughout.

Most women would prefer a drug-free labour, but it's impossible to predict how you'll react to the pain, as every labour is different. But whatever happens, knowing what pain relief is available if you need it, and understanding what interventions may be necessary for the safety of you and your baby, will help you approach the birth with confidence.

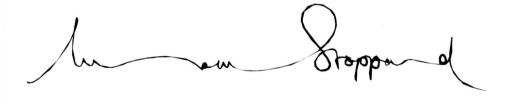

Chapter 1

Choosing the birth you want

These days it's possible to plan exactly the kind of birth experience you want. Your carers will do their best to accommodate your wishes, as well as offer medical care when needed.

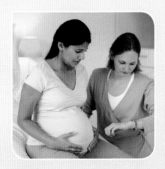
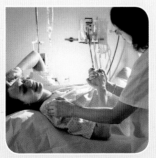
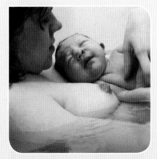

Weight gain and pregnancy

There is no place for any kind of dieting in pregnancy because food restriction nearly always results in the exclusion of essential nutrients.

However, no-one would advocate too great a gain in weight and the old adage "eating for two" is certainly inappropriate.

Most authorities would advise eating to satisfaction and no more. All else being equal, most weight gain takes place in the middle trimester. Little weight increase is experienced in the first. About 0.5–1 kilogram (1–2 pounds) is gained weekly from months four to eight, and less in the ninth month, so that, on an average at least, a total of 11.5 kilograms (26–28 pounds) is gained. This extra weight is split roughly into 2.75–3.5 kilograms (6–8 pounds) for the baby and 6.5–9 kilograms (14–20 pounds) for the baby's support system (you). This weight includes the placenta, amniotic fluid, increased breast tissue, body fat accumulated for milk, enlarged uterus, and extra blood volume.

Looking after yourself

During pregnancy, every organ in your body works harder than normal and uses more energy than before. In addition, your diet must supply all the new materials for your baby's growth. To cope with these high demands, you'll find your appetite increases, you may even experience food cravings that, in most cases, compensate for nutritional deficiencies, and your calorie intake will increase. This is normal. The rule is to eat well and healthily, being careful that your diet also contains all your nutritional requirements. Eat the most varied diet possible and you won't go far wrong. But there are specific pregnancy needs you also have to consider.

Eating well

As a general rule, you can increase your calorie intake by about 200–300 calories a day. Instead of eating two or three main meals a day, try spreading your food intake into five or six smaller meals so that your blood sugar doesn't dip between meals. This will help avoid energy lows and morning sickness in the first three months.

Carbohydrates These provide the essential fuel that gives you energy. Most of your calories should come from carbohydrates, but rather than sugar-based ones you should eat complex unrefined carbohydrates in the form of whole grains, wholemeal bread, porridge, brown rice, potatoes, peas, and beans and lentils, because these provide long-lasting energy and fibre.

It is now well known that the closer your food is to its natural state, the better, so avoid processed carbohydrates where possible. However, simple carbohydrates are absorbed by the system in minutes, so the sugar from fructose (fruit), lactose (milk), and dextrose (honey) is good for a quick energy boost and can help to relieve morning sickness.

Protein This provides the building blocks to enable all your baby's tissues – bone, muscle, cartilage, and blood – to grow, so you should eat at least 100 grams (4 ounces) of protein a day if you can. You may not necessarily eat red meat very often (or at all), but during pregnancy it is important because red meat is a good source of animal protein and the most concentrated source of iron (see p. 9). For vegetarians, milk (skimmed), yogurt, cheese, and eggs are excellent sources of protein, as are seeds, nuts, peanut butter (although high in calories), and the vegetable protein in peas, beans, and lentils. Most bread is protein-enriched. Eat as much fish as you can – it's easily digested pure protein, rich in minerals and vitamins, and oily fish also contains essential fatty acids.

Vitamins All the vitamins are important for maintaining general good health, but some vitamins such as B and C cannot be stored by the body and a daily intake is required. Some vegetables and fruit contain B vitamins, as do meat, fish, dairy products, grains, and nuts. Vitamin C is provided by fresh fruit and vegetables. Vitamin D is found in fish oils and can also be manufactured by the body; this process is triggered by the action of light on the skin, and most people in the UK require about 40 minutes of sunlight per day to produce adequate amounts. Folic acid is important in the prevention of spina bifida, and supplements should be taken three months before conception and during the first trimester. Avoid liver and liver pâtés because they are high in vitamin A and this can cause problems in pregnancy.

Minerals These are essential for your body to function efficiently. Calcium is needed to build the baby's bones and teeth, a process which starts as soon as you conceive. It is wise to make sure your diet is rich in calcium before you become pregnant. During pregnancy, keep your calcium intake high by including broccoli, dried milk, and tinned salmon with bones in your diet. Leafy green vegetables and dairy products also contain calcium. Remember that vitamin D is needed to promote calcium absorption.

Iron This is vital, not just for your baby, but for your own needs, too. Your own iron level must be kept high throughout pregnancy because your baby uses iron so fast that it is cleared instantly from his blood. He is, so to speak, in a constant iron-deficient state.

If you are iron-deficient when you become pregnant, or become so later on, your doctor will prescribe iron tablets or injections to prevent you from developing anaemia. Eat foods that are rich in iron, including red meat, eggs, and offal (not liver); non-animal sources include haricot beans, apricots, raisins, and prunes.

What foods to avoid

We now know that certain common foods carry potentially harmful infective agents that can be dangerous to vulnerable groups such as infants, pregnant women, and the elderly. The chances of your being infected in pregnancy are low but it is best to observe some safeguards.

Listeria This is a rare bacterium found in liver, undercooked meat, cooked, chilled food, and products containing unpasteurized milk, such as soft cheese. Avoid these foods as infection during pregnancy may result in miscarriage or stillbirth.

Toxoplasmosis This is caused by a parasite found in cat and dog faeces, and also in raw meat. It can cause birth defects. Always wash your hands after handling a pet and avoid touching its litter tray. Wear gloves while gardening.

Salmonella This is a bacterial infection found in eggs and chicken that causes fever, abdominal pain, and severe diarrhoea. It is killed by thorough cooking of eggs and poultry.

Good for your wellbeing

Regular exercise can benefit you emotionally as well as physically. You can prepare yourself for the months of change ahead and enjoy yourself at the same time.

✳ You will receive an emotional lift from the release of internal hormones, such as endorphins.

✳ The release of tranquillizing hormones following exercise will make you feel more relaxed and contented.

✳ You can improve your self-awareness as you learn how to use your body in new ways.

✳ Backache, constipation, leg cramps, and breathlessness can be alleviated by regular exercise.

✳ Your energy level will be increased.

✳ You will be better prepared for the work of labour.

✳ You can get back your normal body shape more quickly after delivery.

✳ You can make new friends by meeting other mums at antenatal exercise classes.

✳ You can share the exercise routine with your partner or other members of your family.

Keeping fit

Exercising regularly improves your stamina, suppleness, and strength. It will also help you to cope better with the extra strain placed on your body by pregnancy and labour. By exercising and strengthening certain muscles, you can also develop a better understanding of your body's capabilities, as well as learn how to relax, which will help you during childbirth.

Psychologically, exercising counteracts the tendency to feel clumsy, fat, or ungainly, particularly in the last three months. It increases your circulation, and that can help ease tension.

You may find that it is easier and more comfortable to go through labour if you have good muscle tone. Also, many of the exercises taught in antenatal classes, combined with relaxation and breathing techniques, will help you trust your body during labour. Staying in condition during pregnancy also means that you will regain your normal shape more quickly after delivery.

Regular exercise

It may not seem very appealing to incorporate a daily exercise routine into your busy schedule, but it is quite easy to perform many of the exercises recommended during pregnancy while you engage in other activities: pelvic floor exercises (see p. 11), for example, may be performed while brushing your hair or sitting on the bus.

It is better to exercise several times a day in small bouts than to do it all at once and then not do anything for the rest of the day. Normally, half an hour of rest is enough for a woman to restore her energy, but a pregnant woman may need half a day to recover completely from fatigue. So choose an activity that will be both enjoyable and relaxing.

Recommended activities

Until the last trimester of your pregnancy, you are free to be involved in most sports, as long as you choose something that you have been doing regularly beforehand, and you pursue it regularly once you are pregnant so that your body remains in condition. Some sports and activities are particularly recommended during pregnancy and some should be avoided (see p. 11) at this time.

Swimming This tones most muscles and is excellent for improving stamina. Swimming rarely causes physical injury as your weight is supported by the water, which makes it difficult to strain muscles and joints. Some sports centres offer antenatal water work-out classes.

Yoga Yoga can provide multiple benefits, such as increasing suppleness and reducing tension. It can also teach you to control your breathing and improve your concentration during labour, which is very useful. Always inform your instructor about your pregnancy before taking any classes.

Walking Even if you are not usually an active person, you could at least take up regular walks of a mile or more. Walking is good for your digestion, your circulation, and your figure. Try to walk tall, with your buttocks tucked under your spine, your shoulders back, and your head up. In the last months of your pregnancy, however, your pelvic joint ligaments soften so much that you may find yourself getting a backache if you walk more than a short distance. Always wear well-cushioned, flat shoes.

Activities to avoid

It is best to avoid certain sports such as skiing and horseback riding during pregnancy, because the chances of falling are high, and once you get big, your balance is thrown off by the new weight in front. Other activities, including those listed below, should also be avoided because they put your body under unnecessary stress.

Jogging Don't jog while you're pregnant; it's very hard on your breasts (which need extra support during pregnancy) and it jolts your back, spine, pelvis, hips, and knees.

Sit-ups Any exercise that pulls on the abdominal muscles is a bad idea. The longitudinal muscles of the abdomen are designed to separate in the middle to allow room for the enlarging uterus, and sitting straight up from a lying position encourages them to part even further. The strain may slow down the recovery of abdominal tone after delivery. Leg lifts while you are on your back can have the same effect. To sit up from a lying position, always roll over on to your side and use your arms to push yourself up.

Pelvic floor exercises

The pelvic floor muscles form a funnel that supports the uterus, bowel, and bladder, and serves to close the entrances to the vagina, rectum, and urethra.

During pregnancy, an increase in progesterone causes the muscles to soften and relax. These exercises will help you to keep the pelvic floor well toned and to prevent later problems.

Pull up and tense the muscles around your vagina and anus, as if you were stopping the flow of urine. Hold as long as you can without straining. Relax. Repeat this as often as you can every day.

You should restart this exercise as soon as you can after delivery to minimize the risk of any kind of prolapse. Early exercise will tone up the vagina for sexual intercourse, too. Make it part of your daily routine.

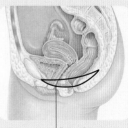

Pelvic floor

The pelvic floor This consists of muscles and fibrous tissue suspended like a funnel from the pelvic bones. It surrounds the urethra, vagina, and anus, with the thickest layer at the perineum.

The case for home birth

A planned home birth can be one of the safest ways you can give birth.

A British report concluded that although 94 per cent of all births take place in hospitals, they are no safer, and may be less safe, than home births.

In Australia, a study of 3,400 home births found that there was a lower perinatal mortality rate, and less need for Caesareans, forceps, and suturing for an episiotomy or a tear, than in hospital deliveries. The mothers were not all "low risk": the group included 15 multiple births, breech deliveries, women who had had Caesareans, and women with previous stillbirths. The group as a whole was older than the national average. Less than 10 per cent of the study group needed to transfer to hospital.

Understanding your choices

Over the past few decades, women have been taking greater control of their own health. In many cases, members of the medical profession have responded enthusiastically to the changing desires and needs of women, and our choices in childbirth have never been greater, nor our wishes more paramount. Today, most women ask to have their children more naturally, and this option should be available to all of them, whether the birth is at home or in hospital. But women shouldn't ignore the benefits a managed birth can provide, particularly when childbirth doesn't go as smoothly as expected.

The modern natural birth

It seems a paradox that you have to request a natural birth, but even today you may find that childbirth is still dominated by obstetricians and a few old-fashioned midwives. However, if you make your preferences known early, a natural birth can be anticipated.

It is reasonable for women to want to have a natural birth, in which there is no fear because the whole process of birth and delivery is familiar; where there is no unnecessary medical intervention; where there is a calm, homely atmosphere; where mothers are allowed to do anything they desire – to take up any positions they find most comfortable – and not be under pressure to take pain-relieving drugs. Female bodies are well designed for giving birth: all the soft tissues of the birth passage can open up so that the baby is gently squeezed out. But breathing and relaxation techniques can make birth even easier to manage, and a number of natural childbirth philosophies advocate these techniques.

Although there are individual differences, all birth philosophies share one common aim – to enable women to give birth in the way they want. Most natural childbirth philosophies include some sort of psychological re-learning to help reduce your expectation of pain and raise your pain threshold. They emphasize the need for intense concentration on breathing patterns and the learned ability to relax the body at will. The best way to experience a totally natural birth is in a dedicated centre or at home.

The modern managed birth

This type of birth (high-tech birth in hospital) came out of a justified concern for the mother and baby, and from increased medical knowledge of the physiological aspects of birth. In a managed birth, labour is actively controlled so that it fits into what is perceived as being normal (this perception can differ, however, depending on the hospital and the obstetrician).

A managed labour is the norm for most hospital births and it is essential for some women who may have complications during pregnancy, labour, and birth – an anticipated breech birth, for example. You will attend antenatal clinics in hospital, and you may well be seen by different doctors and midwives at each visit.

In this setting, you are most likely to experience medical intervention involving some of the most modern procedures in obstetrics. With this kind of labour, epidural anaesthesia is literally on tap and electronic fetal monitoring is standard. Your attendants will notice very small changes in your baby's condition and may be pressured to act on them. Consequently, with this type of birth, there are more inductions and Caesareans, and more frequent use of forceps and ventouse.

Although these practices are beneficial to a percentage of births where intervention is necessary, the routine use of them often cannot be justified by hard evidence, so women who want to have complete control over their deliveries may feel very strongly about their use (see pp. 64–65). Other women clearly believe a hospital setting makes childbirth the event they expect it to be, and would feel cheated, nervous, or even second-class if they didn't have an obstetrician in attendance with high-tech equipment available close by.

Having a home birth

In many European countries, healthy women can opt for a home delivery if their pregnancy has been straightforward. In the UK, it is more difficult. When considering a home birth, most doctors would like you to have had one normal child by a normal delivery before agreeing to a home birth for a second baby. Arranging a home birth can be difficult (see column, right), and you must be very sure that it is the best option for you. Keep an open mind about transferring to a hospital if your labour does not progress well.

Arranging a home birth

Arranging a home birth isn't always straightforward, but if it's what you want it's worthwhile to try.

* Visit your doctor and request a home birth.

* If your doctor agrees, arrange antenatal visits.

* If your doctor says no without a solid medical reason, find a midwife by contacting your hospital or the Independent Midwives' Association (see Useful addresses p. 92).

* Arrange antenatal visits as usual with your new carer.

Water birth and your baby

If you choose to use a birthing pool during your labour, you may worry that your baby will drown if he is actually born under water.

As long as your baby is not kept under water for more than a few moments, he is safe while he is still receiving oxygen from the placenta. Most newborns make strong, vigorous movements of their own accord, and while these may bring them to the surface, you should immediately lift your baby so that his body is clear of the water, to stimulate him to gasp for breath, and give him a welcoming cuddle.

Risks Your doctor may tell you that a home birth is not safe, that it presents too many risks. But there is always some risk attached to giving birth, and statistics have proved that in some circumstances a hospital birth can actually be less safe than a planned home birth (see p. 12). However, unplanned out-of-hospital births can be extremely dangerous, whether it is a teenager trying to conceal an unwanted pregnancy, or a couple whose baby is born en route to the hospital.

Water birth

Over the last few decades, the use of water during labour has gained steadily in popularity. Dr Michel Odent was one of the first obstetricians in the West to offer labouring mothers the use of a shallow birth pool where they could relax when their contractions were at their height. At first, it was never intended that the baby would be born under water but sometimes, by chance, the birth occurred while the mother was in the pool.

Birthing pools are an aid to pain relief; the birth itself isn't necessarily under water, as many people have come to believe. There can be some danger to the baby if he is delivered under water and the head is not lifted out right away (see column, left), and water births must always be supervised by a qualified attendant.

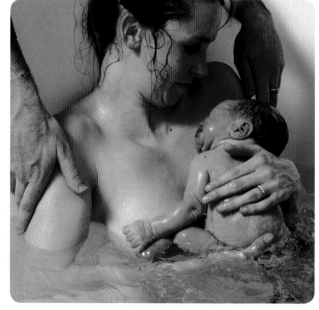

Birth in water Using a birthing pool during labour can help to relax you and reduce the pain of contractions. You are much less likely to be subjected to interventionist procedures because of an imposed time limit. This in turn means that you will have the time required for your tissues and muscles to open and stretch. Your partner can share in the intimacy of a water birth, and your baby can be welcomed with a skin-to-skin cuddle from both of you immediately afterwards.

Many hospitals now offer birthing pool facilities, and there are a few companies that have portable pools for hire (see Useful addresses, p. 92). These can be taken to hospital, if your hospital agrees, or used at home.

Active birth

An active birth is basically one in which you are not in bed and you don't lie down for delivery – you're active. In the past, when the supervision of labour rooms and childbirth were women's responsibilities, mothers were free to move about as they wanted, and to take up any position for birth that they found comfortable. However, once doctors took over the delivery room, women were confined to bed and made to lie on their backs because this made obstetrical manoeuvres easier.

Today, however, the balance has shifted back the other way, and women are rediscovering more natural and mechanically efficient postures for labour and birth. Mothers, supported by partners, are now encouraged to move about and adopt positions that feel comfortable.

Preparation for an active birth is now incorporated in certain childbirth classes, as it has been proven that movements and positions that enable the uterine contractions to be aimed downwards, thus pushing the baby towards the floor, make labour easier and more efficient. A mother who is free to move around may also reduce the need to have an episiotomy, a forceps delivery, or a Caesarean section performed. Moreover, it has been shown that lying on the back can prolong labour and result in other complications (see p. 64).

Partner-assisted birth

Every woman going into labour should have with her someone other than medical and nursing professionals to offer support and encouragement. The best assistant is your partner, especially if he has attended your antenatal classes with you and knows how to help you through each stage of labour.

However, it doesn't have to be your partner. Your mother, sister, or best friend would be an excellent choice, particularly if she's had children of her own and can stay calm if things don't go quite as planned. Whoever you choose should be someone that you trust to make decisions on your behalf, if necessary, so make sure they know your views inside out.

The role of endorphins

The body's natural narcotics, endorphins are usually produced in enormous quantities during labour.

Endorphins are small protein molecules produced by cells in the body. They have a chemical structure similar to morphine and act as pain-reducing chemicals at specific sites in the brain, spinal cord, and all of the nerve endings. In addition, endorphins are thought to be involved in controlling the body's reaction to stress, regulating contractions of the intestinal and uterine walls, and determining mood.

Every person has a unique endorphin response, which probably has a bearing on how different women handle the pain of giving birth.

In most women, the endorphin response appears to "switch on" at a certain point during childbirth, and from then on labour will be arduous, but bearable.

Your experience

If you are giving birth at home, pre-labour (see p. 36) will shift imperceptibly into full labour, without changes in location or attendants.

✳ As there will be no need to travel while in labour, you will continue to remain in the familiar surroundings of your home.

✳ Once your labour starts, notify your midwife. She will come to your house and stay with you throughout.

✳ You will be free to move around and take up any position that feels comfortable.

✳ You will be able to take your own time during labour.

✳ Your membranes will usually be left to rupture spontaneously.

✳ You'll be encouraged to cope with the pain naturally (see p. 42), although pain medication, such as pethidine, can be made available if arranged with the midwife in advance.

✳ Your midwife will try her best to help you retain an intact perineum, thus avoiding an episiotomy.

✳ Your partner and family can be part of the birth.

✳ You will have your baby with you at all times.

✳ After the birth you will be free to celebrate as you wish.

Home birth

The main difference between a home and a hospital birth is that at home the birth is your responsibility and you lead the way. You are the team captain and everyone else is there to support you. The major drawback is that if anything does go seriously wrong, medical back-up will not be immediately available – although the chances of this happening are very small because of the relaxed environment.

The "birthing" room should be properly prepared in advance with your midwife's guidance (in particular, make sure it is warm if the weather is cold), and the necessary supplies should be ready (see p. 28).

What to expect

During the early stages of labour, you will probably find that it is more comfortable if you move around. Many women feel a burst of energy and some get an overwhelming urge to clean the kitchen or sort out a cupboard. This is an expression of the nesting instinct and is a subconscious urge to prepare for the imminent birth. Use this time to arrange your birthing room, gathering sheets and newspapers and getting ready all the things you, your midwife, and the baby will need. Once labour has become established, you or your partner should phone the midwife if she isn't already on her way, as well as any other people you want to be present.

Your midwife will be with you throughout your labour and she will monitor the baby's heartbeat every five minutes with a Sonicaid. She and your partner will encourage you and help you into the most comfortable positions (see pp. 48–49); some pain relief (usually gas and oxygen) will be available if you need it.

As the baby is being born you will probably find it helpful to squat. Your partner may "catch" the baby before putting him to your breast and your baby may breastfeed immediately. The cord will be clamped and cut once it has stopped pulsating, your baby will be quickly checked over (Apgar score, see p. 62), and the midwife will help you deliver the placenta. The baby will be given a thorough examination and weighed on a spring scale.

After this, you will be cleaned up and, if necessary, sutured. Then you will be ready to enjoy your new family member and celebrate together.

The advantages

There are certain advantages to having your baby at home, such as being in familiar surroundings with all the privacy you require. Your partner can play an integral part in the birth and your other children may also be present. You will have the major say in your labour, avoiding routine medical intervention. You won't have to perform according to preconceived medical ideas of what is normal. You will have the same midwife throughout and you will not be separated from your baby or your partner afterwards. You will also avoid the risk of cross-infection from medical staff and other mothers.

The disadvantages

Rest assured that the vast majority of home births proceed without a hitch. However, if something does go seriously wrong, you will have to go into hospital. Your midwife will always accompany you.

There are three main problems that can occur – your baby may have problems being born, he may have difficulties breathing at birth (although this is often due to pain-killing drugs – one risk that does not usually occur at home), and you may have a retained placenta. Not all of these problems are emergency situations. Most breathing difficulties can be eased by clearing the airways, giving oxygen, and a massage. All midwives carry oxygen just in case.

Your baby's experience

Your baby will benefit from the relaxed atmosphere at home and will have exactly the same care from your midwife as if he'd been born in hospital.

* Your baby's heart rate will be monitored by a fetal stethoscope or a hand-held Sonicaid.

* He will emerge into the skilled hands of the midwife, or be "caught" by your birth partner.

* Once breathing, he will be given to you immediately after his birth, and he may suckle spontaneously.

* His umbilical cord will be clamped, and cut once it has stopped pulsating.

* The skin-to-skin contact he experiences as you give him a welcoming cuddle may help his breathing.

* He will be weighed and examined by the midwife but there will be no hurry to clean him up.

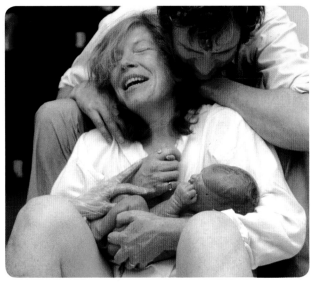

Birth at home Your baby's birth will be a private celebration as he is born into the intimate environment of his family. The absence of bright lights and noise will allow you to greet your baby calmly and gently. If you have other children they can get to know this new member of the family immediately and they can be present at the moment of birth if you wish.

Hospital birth

Most babies are born in hospital. Although more women are choosing to have babies at home, the majority of them, encouraged by their medical advisers or their own predilections, give birth in a hospital. Most hospitals are now paying more attention to the mother's wishes, so there's no reason why you shouldn't enjoy giving birth to your baby in a hospital setting.

What to expect

The unfamiliarity of hospital surroundings can add to the drama of the occasion but here are some tips on making the experience more pleasurable. You will probably have been advised to leave all valuables at home, and trading your own clothes for a hospital gown can feel de-personalizing so, if this bothers you, find out beforehand if you can wear your own nightdress or nightshirt. If you wear contact lenses, ask about the hospital's policy because they may prefer you to bring in a pair of spectacles. If you prefer not to get into bed right away, make it clear that you wish to be able to walk about as necessary.

After admission On arrival, your doctor or midwife will ask you about the progress of labour – the frequency of contractions, and whether your waters have broken, for example. Then a member of the obstetrics team (usually the midwife) will examine your abdomen to confirm the situation, the baby's position will be felt, and the baby's heart checked. Your blood pressure and temperature will be taken and you may be given an internal examination to see how far your cervix has dilated. Fetal monitoring equipment is often then set in place. It can be difficult to move once the equipment is set up, so make sure you are comfortable before you start.

Giving birth If you wish to manage without drugs for as long as possible during labour, the midwives will usually be more than happy to help you cope using other methods (see p. 44). Pain relief with drugs, however, is available and you can ask for smaller doses if you don't feel you need the full measure.

Once the baby is descending, you can ask to be helped into a semi-reclining or squatting position. An episiotomy (see p. 65) is occasionally performed as the baby's head is crowning. Forceps delivery always necessitates an episiotomy but delivery by ventouse may not (see p. 74). Your baby will be delivered on to your abdomen or handed to you to hold so that you can take your first look at each other. Unless you ask not to have it, you will be given an injection of syntometrine into your thigh so that your uterus contracts, helping to expel the placenta.

Your baby will then be assessed by a method called an Apgar score (see p. 62) to make sure she is fit and healthy while you are cleaned up. You are usually sutured by the attending midwife at this point, although in some hospitals you may have to wait for a doctor to do it.

The advantages

In certain situations, a hospital birth offers the best chance of a happy outcome. It is the birth of choice if, for example, you suffer from a medical condition such as heart disease or diabetes, if you are expecting twins, if your baby is known to be breech, or if, as a first-time mother, your obstetrical history just presents too many unknown factors.

Should anything go wrong in hospital, emergency medical assistance will be at hand, and pain medication during labour is readily available. You may feel more confident knowing that your baby can be given immediate treatment in a special care baby unit if the need arises. By staying in hospital after the birth you may be able to have a more complete rest, which could be difficult to arrange at home.

The disadvantages

Once you enter hospital it's easy to feel overpowered by the atmosphere, although some labour wards are becoming more relaxed and if you already know your midwife this is less of an issue. Bear in mind that everybody in hospital is following rules and routines and that you're going to have to fit in with them. That doesn't mean, however, that you have to do anything you aren't happy about. Your partner may feel in the way and even excluded from the birth of his child, so try to include him in whatever way you can.

Your baby's experience

Your baby will be born in a unit supported by medical staff with the expertise to handle any problems that arise.

* An electrode may be attached to the baby's scalp to measure her heart rate during labour.

* With the exception of epidural anaesthesia, the baby will experience any drugs that you are given, and this may mean that she feels drowsy or is slower to feed once she is born.

* She will be handed to you to cuddle and get acquainted with for a few minutes.

* Her umbilical cord will be clamped and cut as soon as it has stopped pulsating.

* She may have her mouth and nose routinely suctioned to clear them of any mucus.

* She will be weighed and examined by the doctor or midwife.

* She will be returned to you, possibly cleaned and wrapped in a blanket, to begin bonding and breastfeeding.

* At a later time she will be thoroughly examined by a doctor for any abnormalities.

Choosing a hospital

You can get information about the hospitals in your area from your doctor, antenatal clinic, social worker, and friends and acquaintances. However, the best way to find out what a hospital can offer you and whether it is right for you is to visit it and ask questions. Make a list of queries beforehand and make sure you get all of them answered so you can come to a confident and wholehearted decision. Only you can decide what will suit you best.

Types of hospital

Most teaching and district general hospitals provide obstetric care. Specialist doctors are always on duty, so if you run into any complications one would attend to you. Larger centres are usually more experienced in dealing with complicated births.

The smaller midwife-led units tend to be more friendly and flexible with less red tape because there are fewer patients and staff. It's easier to meet the people who can help you in such clinics, and you will be able to arrange a more personalized childbirth, although there may be limited pain relief available.

Visiting your hospital

The first thing to do before deciding on a hospital is to tour some of them with your birth partner. There may be a formal maternity tour, often as part of the hospital's antenatal classes, but if not, ask for a personal tour accompanied by a member of staff who knows the clinic well. If the hospital has a policy of not allowing visitors to see the facilities, ask questions. Keep in mind that if they're rigid in their approach to visitors, they are likely to be equally rigid in their approach to maternity care.

The hospital's approach

Once you have decided, it is a good idea to visit the hospital of your choice again so that you can meet the staff who will be looking after you and become familiar with the delivery room and other facilities.

Discuss with your carers if the services offered are satisfactory. Hospitals are there to serve you, and you do have the right to refuse certain procedures. If the hospital is unwilling to listen to your point of view, and does not meet your expectations, you can arrange for a transfer to a different one, or opt for another type of care, such as a family-centred hospital.

If your midwife is part of a team midwife scheme (see p. 23), she will come into the hospital with you and deliver your baby there; the hospital staff are only rarely involved. All being well, you will be discharged within a few hours and need have little to do with the hospital's routines.

A birthing room

Quite a few hospitals now have birthing rooms that are less clinical and more like your own home, with comfortable chairs, low lighting, soft music, piles of cushions on which you can arrange yourself, even a television, and drinks and snacks available.

The purpose of having a birthing room is to help the mother relax, overcome fears, and relieve tension. A normal routine prior to birth makes for a normal delivery, and once you're in a birthing room you will not be moved unless an emergency occurs that requires immediate attention. This ensures there are no uncomfortable breaks with a jarring change of movement, mood, and surroundings.

In a birthing room you can take up whatever position you want to have your baby in. It's not necessary to lie down for the delivery, or to be surrounded by rather intimidating technological paraphernalia.

For a lot of women, a birthing room is the perfect solution for the birth of their choice. It is a compromise between home and hospital births, as it provides similar surroundings and facilities to home, but with emergency expertise on tap if the need arises.

Maternity care units

Family-centred maternity care is offered by some of the more progressive hospitals and larger medical centres. It is a philosophy aimed at nurturing the family unit during labour and delivery, and after birth. It should offer the optional elimination of certain routine procedures and the addition of others, such as low lighting during delivery, keeping parents and baby together unless separation is medically necessary, rooming-in, and early discharge. However, these practices do vary from hospital to hospital, so find out exactly what is offered before committing yourself.

Questions to ask

Once you have chosen a hospital, find out as much as you can by asking questions.

* Will I be able to wear my own clothes and personal effects (rings, contact lenses, glasses, etc.)?

* Can my partner or friend stay with me throughout?

* Will I be able to move around freely during labour, and give birth in any position I want?

* Will I be able to have the same carers throughout labour?

* Can I bring in my own midwife to attend to me throughout labour?

* Does the hospital have a birthing room? If so, are there any beanbags, stools, and birthing chairs provided?

* Does the hospital offer birthing pools? If not, will I be able to use a hired one?

* What is the hospital policy on pain relief, routine electronic monitoring, and induction?

* What kind of pain relief is available? Is this at all times?

* Will I be able to eat and drink if I want to?

* What is the hospital policy on procedures such as episiotomies, Caesareans, and the expulsion of the placenta?

* What is the hospital policy on the separation of parents and child in the first hour or later?

Your attendants

There are many different approaches to birth, so ask your GP, obstetrician, or midwife the following questions to find out exactly what you can expect from him or her:

✳ What are your views on inducing labour?

✳ Under what circumstances would you consider it necessary to rupture the membranes?

✳ Do you believe electronic fetal monitoring is a valuable aid in every birth?

✳ Would you be concerned if my labour progressed more slowly than normal?

✳ What are your views on moving about, the use of water or a birth pool, and breathing techniques to help relieve pain? What drugs do you normally give to control pain?

✳ Would you be concerned if the lights were dimmed during my labour and delivery?

✳ How often do you perform episiotomies during delivery?

✳ Are you happy if I prefer to stand or squat to deliver my baby?

✳ Under what conditions would you consider a Caesarean section to be necessary?

✳ Will we be able to have some time alone with our baby immediately after his birth?

Who will look after you?

There are a number of options open to you regarding who attends your labour – it does not have to be a straight choice between hospital expertise or a home midwife. Wherever you decide to have your baby, the system can usually be tailored to suit your needs.

Your doctor

Your general practitioner will probably be the first professional person that you see. You need to establish his or her views on birth – especially if you are interested in having a home birth. A few doctors are happy to attend a home delivery of a normal pregnancy, many are not so willing, and some fall somewhere in between, preferring you to have at least one straightforward delivery in hospital first. Many doctors provide antenatal care if you are having the baby in the hospital to which they have referred you – try to explore all of the options.

Obstetricians

An obstetrician is a doctor who specializes in medical problems to do with pregnancy and childbirth. When you book into a hospital, you will be assigned to an obstetric consultant and team. You can ask to be referred to a particular obstetrician, but that consultant is not obliged to take you. Although in the past obstetricians tended to be male, there are now more obstetricians who are women – if you feel strongly that you want a woman obstetrician, check whether your hospital employs any. If it does, you should make your preferences clear on your birth plan. There is, however, no guarantee that the obstetrician of your choice will be on duty when you go into labour. You will be unlikely to see your consultant unless you have problems in your pregnancy.

Midwives

Most routine care is provided by junior doctors working with midwives. The modern midwife is a specialist in childbirth, qualified to take responsibility for you before, during, and after the birth. She is able to support and understand you during labour and delivery, and knows when to call for obstetric advice and assistance. Unlike the obstetrician, her focus is on the normal, not the abnormal.

Team midwives Midwives who are a part of the team midwife scheme provide a more personal service. One of a team of midwives is allocated to you and may come to your house when your labour starts, and go to the hospital to deliver your baby; the hospital staff are only rarely involved. If all goes well, you are usually discharged within a few hours into her care.

Hospital midwives Some midwives choose to stay within the hospital and don't go into the community. They often have senior roles in the antenatal or postnatal wards, or in the labour ward.

Independent midwives These midwives provide continuous care in a variety of situations. They will deliver your baby wherever you choose, whether at home or in hospital, and undertake to be with you throughout the labour and delivery. Because your midwife will be your primary caregiver, you will need to get to know her quite well. You may like to ask the following questions:
* What training and experience has she had?
* Does she work alone or with other midwives? Will you be able to meet them?
* What are her considerations in managing labour?
* What is her back-up system? Does she work closely with any particular doctors?
* What equipment, drugs, and resuscitation equipment for the baby does she carry?
* What antenatal care does she provide? Will she visit you at home?
* Under what conditions would she transfer you to a hospital?
* What are her fees?

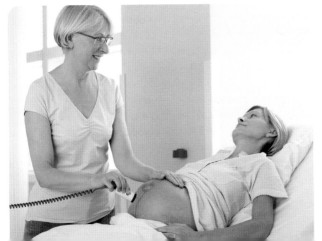

Your birth attendant The professional attendant who assists you should be able to give you the kind of support that you and your partner need, and help you to work with your body to bring a new life into the world.

Your first visit

On your first visit to the antenatal clinic, you will be asked various questions on the following subjects:

✳ Your personal details and circumstances, including age, marital status, next of kin, and religion.

✳ Childhood illnesses or serious illnesses you have had.

✳ Serious illnesses that run in your family or in your partner's family.

✳ Whether there are twins in your family.

✳ What symptoms of pregnancy you have, and the state of your general health.

✳ Details of previous births, pregnancies, or problems in conceiving.

✳ Whether you are taking any prescription medication or whether you suffer from any allergies.

✳ Your menstrual history – when you started, how long your average cycle is, how many days you bleed, and the date of your last menstrual period (LMP).

From the above information, your estimated delivery date (EDD) will be calculated.

Antenatal care

To ensure a healthy pregnancy, you must attend your antenatal check-ups regularly. Although most pregnancies proceed normally, these visits and investigations are vital to monitor your progress and spot problems before any harm is done.

Women at high risk of complications during pregnancy, and women with an existing condition, such as diabetes or having a Rhesus negative blood group, are carefully monitored so that the baby's welfare is never in jeopardy.

The antenatal clinic

You will attend an antenatal clinic either at the hospital where you will have your baby or at your doctor's surgery. Most women attend once a month up until week 32, then every two weeks up to 36 weeks, and then once a week for the last month.

You will need to attend more frequently if any complications develop, such as if you're expecting more than one baby, if you have a pre-existing medical condition, or if you are at risk for any other reason.

Attending an antenatal clinic in a hospital can be intimidating and frustrating: there may be a large number of staff coming and going, and you might be kept waiting for some time. Negative feelings can be made much worse by the discontinuity of care – it's quite possible that you will see different midwives and doctors at every visit. Much of this can be avoided if you opt for shared care, where you mainly see your GP or your midwife for check-ups, with occasional visits to the hospital antenatal clinic.

When you go, try to make the best of your time at the antenatal clinic by taking along something to read or to do, and some food and drink just in case you feel hungry while you are there. Take a friend or your partner with you for company and moral support.

Ideally, your partner should attend at least one antenatal clinic with you so that he can understand what you are going through, and can sympathize with you. He can also have his questions answered and, most importantly, give you moral support.

If you already have young children, arrange for them to be looked after elsewhere if at all possible, because they can be quite a handful in a clinic with little to interest them.

Talking to your carers

Antenatal clinic visits do not usually offer sufficient time for mothers to talk to their carers. However, finding out what alternatives are open to you and discussing your preferences, as well as being reassured about any worries and fears you may be feeling, are very important aspects of your antenatal care, so be prepared to stand up for yourself and insist on extra time to discuss things.

There are always subjects on which you will need reassurance, and so will your partner. No question is too silly to ask, so don't hold back. You and your partner could draw up a list of questions and write them down before your visit. Ideally, your partner should accompany you so that you can ask your questions together.

Your file

At your first antenatal visit all the details of your past medical and obstetric (if any) history, including your menstrual history, will be noted in your file or booklet. This file goes with you wherever you go and the contents can be transferred from one set of case notes to another so that all your carers have important information at hand and continuity of care is assured. In addition, remember to take the file with you to the hospital when you go into labour.

The details on your file or booklet may be difficult for you to understand as many of the medical terms are abbreviated. If you can't make any sense of it, don't hesitate to ask your midwife or doctor for an explanation.

What happens

Your first antenatal visit is the longest because it involves history-taking (see p. 24), which is not necessary on subsequent visits. At each visit your urine is tested for the presence of glucose, protein, or ketones, any of which could indicate a potential problem. Your blood is tested to establish your blood group and your haemoglobin (red cell) levels, which show whether you need iron supplements. Your blood pressure is recorded. At each visit, your abdomen is checked to establish the height of your womb (fundus); this gives the baby's size. Ultrasound scans at about 12 weeks and 18–20 weeks provide an accurate picture of how your baby is growing. If there are any concerns, you may be scanned more frequently. Later on, the baby's heart is checked as well.

Antenatal classes

These classes provide a relaxed and informal setting where you can learn about the techniques of childbirth with other parents-to-be.

It is now accepted that women who are thoroughly prepared for labour and birth are less apprehensive and therefore less tense when they go into labour, which usually results in a less painful and certainly less frightening experience.

However, while classes are primarily meant to prepare you for the birth and to teach you breathing and relaxation techniques useful during labour, they're essential for your birth partner or coach, too. A clear understanding of the stages of labour will enable him or her to give you the help and support you need. No man need feel shy about attending – there'll be other men present at the fathers' classes, and their role at the birth is pivotal for women.

It is also a good idea for both you and your partner to learn about bottle-feeding the baby and to pick up nappy-changing tips at the classes, as well as practising massage techniques for pain relief.

It's your choice

Looking at all the possibilities will help you approach your labour with confidence. Don't feel that it has to be totally managed or completely natural; it can be a blend of many things. Here are some alternatives:

✳ Hospital or home birth.

✳ Partner allowed in for certain procedures, or throughout.

✳ Medical induction of labour or spontaneous start.

✳ Amniotomy (see p. 65) or spontaneous rupture of membranes.

✳ Fetus monitored electronically or manually by Sonicaid.

✳ Confined to bed in first stage of labour or free to move about.

✳ Nothing by mouth, or eat and drink as desired.

✳ Types of pain relief: pethidine, epidural, gas and oxygen, breathing, or diversion.

✳ Catheterization or empty own bladder as necessary.

✳ Commanded pushing or spontaneous pushing.

✳ Deliberate breath-holding or no deliberate breath-holding.

✳ Passive position or active position of your own choice.

✳ You do not touch the vaginal area or the baby's head as he crowns.

✳ Natural expulsion of placenta or use of syntometrine.

Your birth plan

Making a plan for your baby's birth will help to make sure that you are actively involved in the way he is born and in what happens to you as a family after the birth. By carefully considering all your preferences, and by discussing them with your birth attendants and partner, you will be able to establish a bond of trust and so create a happier and more comfortable birth environment.

A consensus plan

Think about the issues that are important to you and then find out whether what you want is feasible. There is no point in making a plan that cannot be used once you are in labour. You should discuss your plan with your GP early in your pregnancy so that he or she can refer you to a consultant obstetrician most likely to accord with your wishes. You should make specific enquiries about the routines used where you intend to give birth, because some hospitals will not be able to meet your requirements. Discuss these with your antenatal teacher and others involved in your antenatal care – they will be able to advise you about the experiences other mothers have had in local hospitals and with particular doctors.

Hospital response Your hospital team may be pleased to see how well you have prepared yourself for the labour, and your full participation will probably be encouraged. Some mothers have experienced negative reactions from hospital staff on the grounds that a birth plan may interfere with their standard practices. Don't be intimidated – just remember that your baby is your responsibility and so is the way in which you give birth.

Working together Co-operation is an important feature of the birth plan. By working it out in detail with all your attendants, including your partner, you should be able to alleviate any anxieties and feel more in control of your baby's birth. Make sure that the hospital staff also know about your fallback position in case your original plan cannot be followed for any reason. Try to maintain a friendly relationship with your caregivers because they are not bound to follow your wishes. Give a copy of the plan to each of them; a copy should also be put with your hospital records with details of any special needs.

Chapter 2

Getting ready

Whether you have decided on
a home birth or a hospital birth, you
need to **plan** and **prepare** for the event at
least a few weeks before your due date.
Enjoy the preparation – it will help you
feel that you are **providing the ideal
setting** for your delivery.

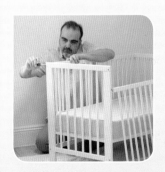
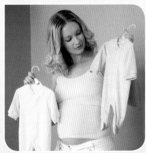
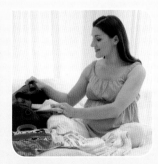

Your pre-labour checklist

Although you can make most of your preparations well in advance, you will still have a few things to take care of at the last minute. When you do go into labour (see p. 38), try to remember the following:

✳ Call your midwife.

✳ Make contact with your partner or birth assistant.

✳ Get in touch with whoever is going to care for your other children, if not your partner.

✳ Check that the birthing room is ready.

✳ Check that your labour aids are conveniently at hand.

✳ Make yourself a hot, sweet drink.

Preparing for a home birth

Once you have decided to go for a home birth, check with your midwife for detailed advice on the preparations you'll need to make. Think about what you will need for a home birth about four weeks in advance of your due date, so that you do not have to rush around getting everything organized at the last minute and you are at least partly prepared if your baby comes early.

Advance preparations

The room you intend to give birth in should be arranged so that it is convenient and comfortable for you. Set the bed at right angles to the wall, with plenty of space on each side so that the midwife has easy access.

Getting the room ready Whether you deliver your baby on to the floor or the bed, the area below and immediately around you will need to be protected during the birth. In order to do this, make sure that you have some old clean sheets, towels, and plastic sheeting ready so that they can be put down when the time comes. Plastic sheeting is available from your local builders' merchant or DIY shop, although an old shower curtain or plastic tablecloth can also be used.

Facilities for your midwife Ideally, your midwife will need a small table or a tea trolley next to the bed, to put her instruments and other equipment on (although a couple of tea

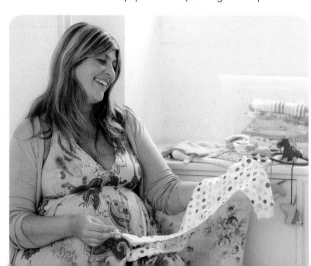

Advance preparations Try to prepare everything you are likely to need well in advance.

trays will do), and a bright, adjustable reading lamp so that she can direct light on to your perineum. A torch (with spare batteries and bulb) would be useful to have at hand in case of a power cut. You should also make sure that you stock up on food and drink a few days before you are due.

When labour starts

When your contractions are coming every 15 minutes, are about one minute long, and don't die away when you move around, it is time to contact your midwife. Although it is common for first labours to take a while to get going, your midwife needs to know that the process has begun. She is likely to advise you to try and relax and get some rest until you are in full labour, because it is important to conserve your energy. All independent midwives can be contacted by mobile phone, so it is easy to keep in touch.

Final preparations Make sure everything else that you and the midwife will need, for the birth and immediately afterwards, is prepared and ready to hand – including your comfort aids (see p. 32), bowls for washing, a bedpan (or a clean bucket), clean towels, large plastic bags for the soiled sheets, and sanitary pads. Then put out a clean nightdress or large nightshirt for yourself, air your baby's clothes, and prepare the cot.

Your midwife Her delivery equipment will include a sphygmomanometer to take your blood pressure, Pinard stethoscope or (more usually) a Sonicaid to listen to the baby's heart, Entonox (gas and oxygen) cylinder, urine-testing sticks, local anaesthetic and syringes, scissors, suture material, mucus extractor, resuscitation equipment, intravenous equipment (in case of bleeding), and syntometrine. If you prefer to have pain-relieving drugs such as pethidine on standby, your GP can give you a prescription to collect in advance.

Unexpected hospitalization If a serious problem arises and you have to go into hospital instead of giving birth at home, your midwife or doctor will accompany you. Being unable to have a home birth after all your preparation and anticipation can be disappointing, but this is a possibility you and your partner should consider in advance, so that it will be easier to cope with if it happens.

When not to have a home birth

In certain circumstances a hospital birth is your only option, and going ahead with a home birth would be unwise.

There are a number of factors that can make a hospital birth necessary. Some, such as diabetes, will mean that you have to plan on a hospital delivery; others, such as placental abruption (sudden separation of the placenta), will mean that you have to abandon your plans for a home birth and go immediately to hospital. The following factors also rule out a home birth:

* If your previous pregnancies have been complicated.

* When your pelvis is too small for your baby's head to pass through.

* When your baby is presenting in the breech position.

* When there is a medical condition that puts you, your baby, or both of you at risk, such as high blood pressure, anaemia, diabetes, excess amniotic fluid, active herpes, placenta praevia, placental abruption, or pre-eclampsia.

* When you have a multiple pregnancy.

* When labour is premature.

* When your pregnancy goes well beyond your EDD (see p. 66).

Going to hospital

If you get everything ready and pack the things you will need to take with you to hospital a few weeks in advance, you won't have to worry about being caught unprepared when your labour begins.

What to take

The items you will need with you in hospital fall into three categories: clothes and other personal effects for yourself, clothes and nappies for your baby, and your comfort aids for labour (see p. 32). Contact the hospital to find out what you should bring with you and what it will provide for your baby.

For yourself You will need two or three maternity bras and front-opening cotton nightdresses, a quantity of breast pads, a dressing gown and slippers, plenty of pants, and a supply of super-absorbent sanitary towels (these may be provided by the hospital). Pack an overnight bag with your usual toiletries, as well as shampoo, a couple of towels and face cloths, a hairbrush, a small mirror, make-up, face cream, and tissues. If you have drawn up a birth plan (see p. 26), remember to take it with you.

For your baby If the hospital does not provide nappies and baby clothing for your stay, you will need to take them with you. Take vests, nightdresses or stretchsuits, a shawl, a hat, and a blanket to wrap your baby in when you go home.

Is it time?

As you approach your estimated delivery date, your body will begin to give you signals that it is preparing for the birth. You may experience the symptoms of pre-labour (see p. 36) and,

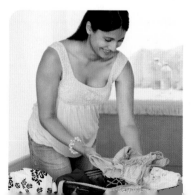

Getting ready Make sure that you have everything ready and packed well in advance.

in some cases, labour. Although you don't have to rush to hospital when any of the following occur, you should be prepared for them and make your final preparations. The "show" normally comes first, and either the waters breaking or contractions will follow, although sometimes contractions precede the first two (see pp. 36–37 for an explanation of the early signs).

The "show" A plug of blood-tinged mucus, which had been sealing your cervix prior to birth, becomes dislodged during the early first stage of labour, if not before. It is usually easily recognizable.

The waters break Pressure due to contractions or the baby's head pressing on the membranes of the amniotic sac may cause it to rupture before the start of labour. The amniotic fluid will then escape, either as a trickle or in a rush.

Regular contractions Whether or not you have been aware of any contractions previously, you will start to experience them – in the form of severe cramp-like pains that come at regular intervals and last longer and longer. The interval between contractions gets shorter.

When to go

If, over an hour, you notice that your contractions are coming every 15 minutes, are about one minute long, and don't die away when you move around, call your hospital or midwife according to prior arrangement. At this time, your first level of breathing (see p. 44) will probably no longer be adequate, and you will be getting ready to use different types of breathing patterns. This is when pre-labour is easing into the first stage. There is absolutely no need to rush into hospital because the first stage usually lasts at least eight hours for the first baby. However, if you live a long way from the hospital or are particularly worried about getting there in time, go as soon as you feel that you have to.

Transport You will probably travel to the hospital by car or by taxi. If you plan to go by car, you or the driver should check beforehand that the car is in good condition and there is a full tank of fuel. Do not drive yourself unless there is absolutely no other alternative.

Your journey to hospital

If you are travelling to the hospital by car, try to make sure that your journey will be both safe and comfortable.

In the weeks leading up to the birth, both you and whoever is going to drive you to the hospital should be thoroughly familiar with the route. Find out how long the journey is likely to take at different times of the day, and work out alternative routes in case, on the day, you encounter heavy traffic or other delays. Check to see if you need to take any money for the car park and have the right amount ready. You should also check out the entrances to the hospital and find out how to get from the entrances to the ward – especially during the night.

The car The bigger the car you travel in, the more comfortable you are likely to be. You will probably be more comfortable and safer in the back seat, and if it is large enough, you can lie down rather than sit.

Sudden birth If your baby starts to arrive while you are still on your way to the hospital, try to remain calm. You have a good chance of getting there before the baby is actually born, but if things are moving too fast, it is best to stop the car, phone for an ambulance, and prepare for an emergency delivery (see p. 76).

Comfort aids for labour

When organizing the things you will need for the birth, remember to get ready all the items that will make your labour a more comfortable experience. It's a good idea to prepare your comfort aids in advance, so that you don't forget anything in all the excitement when labour starts, and you won't be caught unprepared if your labour starts sooner than expected.

Provisions for comfort

Your midwife or hospital attendants will give you advice about what comfort aids may be useful during labour. If you're having a home birth, keep all your aids together in your birthing room. If you've opted for a hospital birth, pack them in a bag and keep it next to your hospital case. Make sure your birth assistant also knows where they are kept, so that they are not left behind.

 If you are planning to have an active birth, you may need to take your own large cushions or a bean bag into the hospital with you. These are ideal if you want to sit in a supported squat position in labour and the hospital room contains only a bed.

Distractions In the early stages of labour, before it is really established, it is likely that for quite a long period of time you'll feel that nothing much seems to be happening. It will probably help distract your attention and pass the time if you and your partner have some diversions available, such as magazines, books, playing cards, or a music player (preferably with ear phones). Some women have found that playing soothing music helps set the mood for a relaxed birth.

Keeping cool There will probably be times when you won't want anything to drink, but you would really like something wet and cool in your mouth. You may find it comforting to suck on crushed ice or an ice cube, in which case you will need a portable icebox for storage if you are going into hospital. Alternatively, you may prefer to moisten your mouth by sucking on a small natural sponge that your birth partner has dipped in cold water.

General comfort aids

Your face is likely to become very hot and sweaty, and you will probably find it refreshing to have it mopped with an absorbent face cloth. In addition, your birth partner can create a slight breeze on your face by using a hand-held electric fan.

Keeping warm During the later stages of labour, and particularly immediately after the birth, some women begin to shake quite visibly with cold, so bring along some thick socks in case this happens.

Comfort aids If your hair is long or falls over your face, a few hair grips, slides, combs, or a hairband will help to stop it from irritating you.

Your lips are likely to become very dry because of breathing through your mouth, so include a lip salve that you can rub on to your lips to prevent them from cracking.

If you become nauseous and actually vomit, you will undoubtedly feel much better if you are able to clean your teeth afterwards, so don't forget to take your toothbrush and some toothpaste or, if you prefer, a small bottle of mouthwash.

A box of tissues is useful, as are scented wipes to cleanse the face, neck, and hands. For freshening up, you may want to splash on some eau de cologne.

Don't forget that your partner will need a charged-up mobile phone to tell everyone the news of your new arrival. And, of course, take a camera to record the happy event.

Your partner's comfort aids

Your birth partner may find attending your labour more comfortable if they have certain items set aside for their own use. Here are a few suggestions:

✳ A pack of wipes for freshening face and hands

✳ Snacks and drinks (see p. 34).

✳ Distractions for your other children if they are present

✳ A change of clothing

✳ Charged camera and memory cards, or a video camera if permitted

✳ A mobile phone, to share the happy news

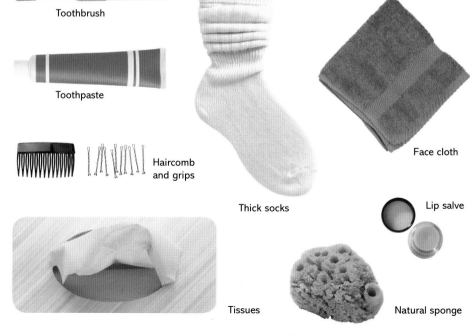

Toothbrush

Toothpaste

Haircomb and grips

Thick socks

Face cloth

Lip salve

Tissues

Natural sponge

Your nourishment

In case your labour starts slowly or is particularly long and tiring, you may need to take some food and drink into the hospital to keep you going during the first stage. Your partner will also need refreshments to keep up his or her energy levels.

✳ Make several sandwiches for yourself and your partner.

✳ Chocolate bars are excellent for providing instant energy.

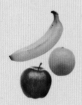

✳ Fresh fruit is refreshing, portable, and a good source of energy.

✳ Sweets can be sucked slowly, and also provide glucose.

✳ Drink diluted fruit juices or cooled water. Fizzy drinks are best avoided.

Relieving discomfort with massage

Many women find that the discomfort of labour, particularly backache, can be alleviated with massage (see p. 44). Counterpressure can be provided by your partner using his hands or a spinal roller, or even a tennis ball! If using the hands to massage, it is best to use a bit of cream, talcum powder, or vegetable-based massage oil to stop your skin from being dragged or rubbed sore. A hot pad placed in the small of your back can also act as a compress to soothe backache.

Food and drink

As a first labour can last up to 14 hours, check whether the hospital's policy allows you to eat during labour. These days it usually does – so pack a few snacks such as chocolate bars, which will give you instant energy. In fact, shortly before labour, the ability of your stomach to absorb food decreases, so you should eat only easily digestible food.

Your partner will certainly need some food to sustain him during your labour and probably won't want to leave your side to go in search of it – especially if it is in the middle of the night – so make sure that you pack a supply of sandwiches, energy bars, and fruit for him, too.

After the birth, you are both likely to want something to eat straight away. You will also need to drink: a bottle or vacuum flask of diluted, unsweetened fruit juice or cold water is ideal for you, although your partner might prefer canned soft drinks.

Pain-relieving items

Occasionally a woman may feel the discomfort of uterine contractions mainly as low back pain. This is usually due to the stretching of the cervix as it dilates, or because your baby lies in the posterior position. These items will be useful to relieve backache during labour:

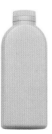

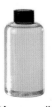
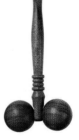

Powder   Tennis ball   Massage oil   Spinal roller

Chapter 3

Birthing begins

After the long wait, it is understandable that you will feel **anxious and impatient** for the **first signs** that labour is under way. This is an exciting moment. There is **hard work and some discomfort** ahead but there are several ways to **relieve pain** that will help you cope.

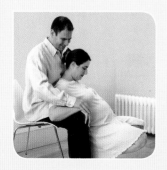 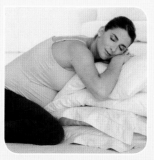 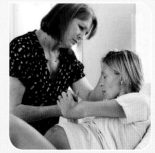

Pre-labour and labour

Medical definitions of labour divide it into three separate stages. During the first stage, the cervix opens out fully to allow the baby to pass through, at the end of the second stage the baby is born, and in the third stage the placenta is delivered. All stages are discussed in detail over the following pages. But, in addition to these three stages, most women will experience pre-labour. Your experience of labour may be much more colourful and exciting than the above definition. Go into it believing that very little can go wrong and very little will go wrong.

Pre-labour

Before real labour begins, hormones secreted by your uterus and the baby prepare your body for birth in a number of ways. During the last few weeks, you will probably notice a few signs of your impending labour. However, just as each woman's experience of labour and birth is unique, so these pre-labour symptoms affect each woman in varying degrees. They provide useful signals that indicate to you that labour is imminent.

Engagement To position himself for the journey through the birth canal, your baby will move lower down so that his presenting part, usually the head, will settle into your bony pelvis. This is known as engagement, and you will experience it as a feeling of lightening. If this is your first pregnancy, engagement will probably occur about two to three weeks before the onset of labour. If you've had previous babies, the baby's head may remain higher until just before labour starts, as your uterine muscles may have stretched, and so will exert less pressure on your baby. You will know when engagement occurs because pressure on your diaphragm eases and breathing becomes easier. On the other hand, you will probably have to pass urine more frequently, as your baby is now pressing down on your bladder.

Braxton Hicks' contractions During your pregnancy, your uterus has been practising for the strong contractions needed during labour with weak, irregular contractions, named after the doctor who first described them. The majority of women feel them throughout the last few months of their pregnancies. If you place your hand on your abdomen, you may be able to feel it hardening and tightening for approximately 25 seconds.

Unlike real labour contractions, these are usually painless, although a few women find them slightly uncomfortable. If you feel any discomfort, sitting down quietly should help to ease it.

Runs of Braxton Hicks' contractions may become more frequent and intense as real labour approaches, helping to prepare the cervix for dilation and to increase the circulation of blood to the placenta. When you feel a run of Braxton Hicks', practise the relaxation techniques you intend to use during labour; the tightening and relaxing of your uterus will give you a good idea of how a contraction feels as it waxes and then wanes.

Some mothers misinterpret Braxton Hicks' as real labour, arriving at hospital only to be told they can go home again. This is known as false labour (see p. 38).

"Nesting instinct" You may experience a surge of energy to make final preparations for the arrival of your baby. If you feel the need to rush around cleaning or decorating the house, or cooking large meals, try to restrain yourself. You will need all this extra energy for coping with labour and delivery.

The show An obvious sign that labour is imminent is the appearance of the show – the plug of mucus that seals your cervix during pregnancy, providing protection against infection. Although the show often does not appear until labour is underway, the cervix may widen enough for the mucus plug to be dislodged up to 12 days before labour begins. This sticky substance may be slightly brown, pink, or blood-tinged from the capillaries that attached it to the cervix. The show signals dilation of the cervix.

Premenstrual feelings Physical and emotional changes similar to those you experience premenstrually may occur. You may also feel crampy, with pressure in your rectum, and feel the need to empty your bowels and pass urine frequently.

What your baby is doing

While no one actually knows for certain why labour starts, when it does, there is evidence to show that the baby plays a major role.

Secreting hormones The onset of labour is triggered by the secretion of hormones – some pregnancy hormone levels drop, others rise. New hormones are secreted, one of which is produced by your baby.

Engagement Throughout your pregnancy, your baby will be floating in his amniotic sac above the pelvic brim. As his birth approaches, his head, or his bottom if he is in a breech presentation, will descend lower down into your pelvis and become engaged.

Kicking less You may notice that he is quieter than in previous months. From time to time you may feel a slight flurry of movement, although if all movement appears to have ceased completely, contact your doctor or midwife immediately.

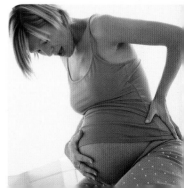

Approaching labour You may be anxious to get your delivery over with, or feel that you aren't ready for labour. This can be an emotional time, so try to stay calm.

Is it false labour?

It's not always easy to distinguish false labour from real labour if it's your first pregnancy. As a general rule, if you're in any doubt, you're not in real labour.

Although false labour is only a rehearsal, try not to be too disappointed; false labour heralds real labour, and you won't have much longer to wait. There are some simple differences between false and real labour:

Regularity False contractions never really settle down and become truly regular.

Frequency Contractions are sporadic. They may vary from 10 minutes to 20 minutes apart, with no steady pattern.

Effect of movement False contractions usually weaken or subside altogether if you get up and move around; real contractions increase.

Strength False contractions do not get progressively stronger. They may even weaken from time to time, and then disappear.

Some women, especially if they are working, or get overtired or overexcited, may slip in and out of false labour for a few days before real labour begins. Talk to your doctor or midwife about the contractions; they will advise and reassure you. Keep on the move, and stay upright to help labour progress.

The first stage

The climax of your pregnancy is going into labour. In medical terms, the first stage begins when your contractions bring about dilation and thinning of the cervix, and ends when effacement (thinning) and dilation (opening) are complete. At this point your midwife will confirm that you are fully dilated. This is the end of the first stage of labour.

What happens in labour

It is difficult to be sure about the onset of labour because it's so different for each woman. However, certain classic signs – intense uterine contractions, dilation and thinning of the cervix, and rupturing of the membranes – are taken to mean that labour is underway.

Contractions When true labour starts, the nature of contractions changes. They become more rhythmical, more painful, and occur at regular intervals. These contractions are not within your control and, once they have begun, will not stop until your baby is born.

You can time your contractions from the beginning of one contraction to the beginning of the next. In early labour, contractions are usually about 30–60 seconds long, at intervals of about 5–20 minutes. This can vary, as some women may not notice their first contractions until they are closer together, say every five minutes. During the active phase, contractions usually last 60–90 seconds, at intervals of 2–4 minutes.

As your uterus tightens, you may feel a sensation of pain, similar to menstrual cramps, spreading around your lower abdomen like a tight band. This is because the uterine muscle becomes short of oxygen as the blood vessels of the wall are compressed. The uterus is a huge muscle that needs a lot of energy during contractions.

Every woman feels contraction pains differently, but in early labour they may be similar to menstrual cramps or mild backache. Some women experience persistent and severe backache (see p. 70).

Very often, a contraction feels like a wave of discomfort right across your abdomen that reaches a peak for a few seconds and then diminishes; at the same time you can feel a hardening and tightening of the uterine muscle, which is held at the peak of its intensity for a few seconds before it relaxes.

The cervix dilates and thins The cervix is usually a thick-walled canal about 2 centimetres (¾ inch) long, and firmly closed. During the last few weeks of pregnancy, hormones should have softened your cervix, but the intense contractions of first-stage labour are needed to dilate and thin it. In the early (latent) first stage, your cervix will dilate very little, then progress to full dilation in the active phase. The pain increases as you become fully dilated. Eventually, the entire cervix opens up and is made one with the uterus, thus creating a continuous channel through which your baby can emerge.

The waters break The membranes of the amniotic sac may rupture painlessly at any time during labour, although this usually occurs towards the end of the first stage. Fluid may leak or gush out; the flow depends on the size and site of the break, and whether or not the baby's head is plugging the hole.

Usually, when the membranes rupture spontaneously near term, labour occurs within a short time, although in a few instances it is delayed – if the baby's presenting part is not engaged, or if the baby is presenting abnormally. Delay also occurs in many normal cases.

How long does labour last?

Every woman's experience of labour is unique, and the time span can't be predicted. However, an average labour lasts about 12–14 hours for first-time mothers, and about seven hours for subsequent labours. If your first labour lasts longer than 12 hours, or nine hours in subsequent labours, your obstetrician may intervene.

The first stage of labour can be regarded as having three separate phases. The early, or latent, phase is the longest, lasting about eight hours for first babies, during which the cervix will soften and you will feel contractions occurring with increasing frequency and length. Try to conserve your energy during this time.

The next, active phase when the cervix is dilating, is shorter, lasting from three to five hours, and this is when your contractions become more painful and you may want pain relief (see p. 42). The final phase of dilation (sometimes called transitional) is the shortest and most intense, usually lasting under an hour, and comes just before you begin to push.

Your cervix dilates

The normally tough cervix must be stretched thin and opened wide before your baby's head can pass through. The contractions of the first stage of labour achieve this.

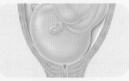

Before labour Your cervix is normally thick and closed but has been softened by hormones.

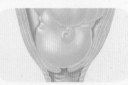

Early (latent) phase Your cervix begins to thin (efface) before it can stretch and dilate.

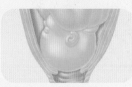

Active dilation When your cervix is about 5cm (2in) wide, it is halfway to full dilation and delivery.

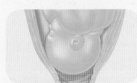

End of the first stage Your cervix is fully dilated when it is 10cm (4in) wide. Now the head can descend.

Your hospital admittance

When you arrive at the hospital, the midwife will prepare you for the birth. There are certain routine examinations that you will have to undergo.

* While consulting your notes, the midwife will ask you questions about your labour's progress – whether your waters have broken and how often your contractions are coming.

* You will be asked to undress and put on a hospital gown or your own T-shirt or nightdress.

* You will then be examined; the midwife will palpate your abdomen to feel the baby's position; she will listen to the fetal heartbeat, take your blood pressure, pulse, and temperature, and give you an internal examination to see how far your cervix has dilated.

* You will be asked to give a urine sample to test for the presence of protein and sugar.

* You may be offered a shower or bath and will be shown to the delivery room. If you have any questions or you want to make your feelings known to the staff, now is the time to remind them of your birth plan.

Hospital procedures

Each hospital has its own set of routine procedures for labour. If you have visited the hospital beforehand, met the staff who will be looking after you, and looked at the labour and delivery rooms, you will have some idea of the hospital routine. Hospitals can seem intimidating but are less so once you get to know them.

Admission to hospital Once you've arrived in hospital you may be offered a wheelchair to transport you from the hospital entrance to the labour ward. If your labour is well advanced, you'll welcome a wheelchair, but if not, you should be allowed to walk if you wish.

You may have outlined in your birth plan (see p. 26) how you wish your labour to go, and once you've met your midwife or doctor, this is the time to make sure they have a copy that you can look over with them. They will also make some checks and will ask you questions about your labour (see column, left and p. 18).

If you aren't happy with any procedure, if equipment, lights, or needles frighten you, or if you are upset by a staff member, make your feelings known at the time. Your birth partner can voice your feelings if you aren't feeling strong enough.

Examinations Your baby's heart will be regularly monitored by fetoscope, Sonicaid, or an electronic fetal monitor (see p. 41). You will probably have an internal examination every four hours during the first stage to check the dilation of your cervix.

Each time you have an internal examination, ask how you are progressing. It is very comforting to know how far your cervix has dilated between examinations. If your birth partner is asked to leave during an internal examination, feel free to say that you would prefer him or her to stay. If you're asked a question while you are having a contraction, concentrate on your relaxation techniques and answer when the contraction is over.

Pain relief After the admission procedures, you will be visited by the anaesthetist if you have opted for some form of medical pain relief (see pp. 42–44). If you are having epidural anaesthesia, the procedure will be set up now. This usually takes 10–20 minutes. The anaesthetist may then leave you with your birth partner and midwife, but will return later to check and top up the anaesthetic. Pethidine, and gas and oxygen are always available.

Electronic fetal monitoring

This high-tech replacement for the ear trumpet is used to track the baby's heartbeat. Electronic fetal monitoring (EFM) will be used routinely in all cases of high-risk pregnancies, but most mothers and babies don't require it. You will have EFM if you are being induced or your labour is being accelerated for any reason, or if you have opted for epidural anaesthesia. Its main function is to give warning of fetal distress.

If your doctors decide that you and your baby would be better off with EFM, try to see it as a source of reassurance. You can watch your baby's heartbeat during labour and know that he is fine.

What it is There are two kinds of electronic monitor, external and internal. An external monitor can be used early in labour and is sometimes used during pregnancy to check the baby's wellbeing. You'll have two belts strapped around your abdomen: one to assess the frequency and strength of the contractions, the other to record the baby's heartbeat. The baby's heartbeat and your contractions are recorded on a cardiotocography (CTG) printout.

Internal monitoring can only be undertaken once your membranes have ruptured or are ruptured for you. A tiny electrode will be clipped onto the baby's head – it gives a slightly more accurate recording of the heartbeat. In some units, in addition to the baby's monitor, a second monitor may be placed between your baby and the uterine wall to measure the pressure and contractions.

During a contraction, blood flow to the placenta is reduced for a few seconds, and your baby's heart rate will dip. This is quite normal and the heart rate returns to baseline when the contraction passes. If the return to baseline is delayed, your baby may be distressed and action can be taken early to protect his wellbeing.

The latest type of EFM, known as telemetry, uses radio waves and allows you to walk around because the baby's monitor is attached to a transmitter strapped to your thigh. The older equipment confines you to a bed or chair.

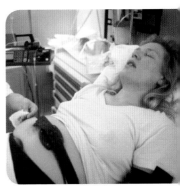

Monitoring in labour Contractions are recorded by an external monitor strapped to your abdomen. An internal monitor is attached to your baby's presenting part, usually the head, by piercing his skin. It provides an electrical contact that picks up his heartbeat. When they are born, some babies' heads will be bruised or have a rash where the electrode was attached.

How drugs affect you

Apart from offering pain relief, drugs can affect your experience of childbirth in other ways. Make sure you opt for the type that will help enhance, rather than detract from, the pleasure of your baby's birth.

Drowsiness This is a common side-effect of gas and oxygen, tranquillizers, and narcotics. Some women enjoy the sensation of drifting, but sometimes this can make mothers feel they lack control. A few women have become so light-headed they were unaware of what was happening around them, and gave birth without realizing it had happened.

Dizziness Pethidine and other narcotics can sometimes induce a feeling of confusion or disorientation, and some mothers have even had hallucinations.

Nausea The sensation of nausea is usually slight with gas and oxygen, but is quite common after using pethidine and other narcotics, and a few mothers may suffer attacks of vomiting.

Your state of mind can have a major effect on the intensity of pain experienced in labour. Excessive tension can affect the uterus, increase your perception of pain, and lengthen labour. So, if the use of drugs will make you less anxious and more relaxed, there is no point in depriving yourself.

Pain relief

For many women, particularly first-time mothers, anticipation of their baby's birth may be overshadowed by worry about pain during labour. Labour invariably involves some level of pain, but you can build up your confidence by preparing for the intensity of contractions, trying to understand your own limits of pain tolerance, and by learning about the different methods of pain relief. View the pain as a positive element of labour – each contraction brings the birth of your baby nearer.

Coping with pain

The kind of pain you'll experience during contractions can vary. It may feel like a thick band being squeezed around your abdomen as the uterus hardens and tightens for several seconds before relaxing. Some women compare it to severe menstrual cramps, others experience backache, but there may be a combination of sensations as the contraction peaks and then subsides.

Individual response You may prefer not to use certain drugs during your labour as they can dim your awareness of what is happening; however, it is very difficult to know the level of pain you can manage without relief, particularly if this is your first baby. Some women are surprised by the overpowering intensity of their contractions, others may find their pain worsens through fear and anxiety. Analgesia, such as epidural anaesthesia, can offer complete relief from pain, while gas and oxygen and narcotics help reduce pain to bearable levels. Many women opt for no drugs in the early part of the first stage, then have gas and oxygen towards transition. Don't be self-critical if you do need drugs for pain relief – it isn't a sign of cowardice. Remember, labour isn't a test, and drugs may even be essential to deliver your baby.

If you wish to participate fully in your baby's birth without dimming your consciousness of the physical and emotional sensations, there are alternatives to drugs for pain relief (see pp. 44–45).

A clear choice Find out as much as possible about the types of pain relief that will be available. Have a discussion with your doctor, midwife, and hospital attendants, and then outline your choices in your birth plan (see p. 26). Be prepared for plans to change if any complications arise.

Pain-relieving drugs

In large hospital units, all the following types of pain relief will be on offer. In midwife-led units or home deliveries only narcotics or gas and oxygen are available.

Regional anaesthetics These remove sensation from a part of your body by blocking the transmission of pain from nerve fibres.

The most widely used form of this type of anaesthesia is the epidural block. This prevents pain from spreading out from your uterus by acting as a "nerve block" in your spine. A well-managed epidural removes all sensation from your waist to your knees, but you remain alert and it does not affect your baby. It is recommended if you have a difficult labour, pre-eclampsia, or severe asthma.

First, a local anaesthetic is given in your back to numb the area for the injection. A fine, hollow needle is then inserted into the epidural space (the region around the spinal cord) and a thin tube known as a catheter is threaded down inside the hollow needle. The needle is removed, leaving the catheter, which is taped in position. Anaesthetic is syringed into the catheter, which is sealed, although it can be topped up at any time if necessary. You need to let your attendants know in advance that you wish to have an epidural because it must be given by a skilled anaesthetist, and it usually takes 10–20 minutes to set up. The anaesthetic will take effect within a few minutes.

A spinal anaesthetic is used as a one-off injection, which numbs the sensation below your waist. It is very similar to an epidural but no catheter is left in place and it cannot be topped up. This is used for Caesarean and forceps deliveries.

To administer a pudendal block, anaesthesia is injected straight into your vagina near the pelvic region, blocking the pudendal nerve. This numbs the lower part of your vagina, and may be used if you have an episiotomy.

How drugs affect your baby

Most drugs will cross the placenta and affect your baby once they are in your bloodstream. Those used in epidural anaesthesia, however, do not enter your baby's blood.

Drowsiness A large dose of sedatives or tranquillizers may affect his ability to suckle and to respond to you immediately after he is born.

Breathing and sucking If you take pethidine late in your labour, it could affect your baby at birth, because narcotics can depress your baby's breathing and make sucking inefficient.

Spinal cord

Catheter

Epidural space

Epidural anaesthetic After an injection of local anaesthetic in your back, a catheter is inserted into the epidural space and the anaesthetic is injected through this.

Ways you can breathe

Relaxing your body and focusing on your breathing will help alleviate your anxiety and let you ride out your contractions. Practise breathing patterns beforehand with your birth partner so that he or she can guide you during labour, if necessary.

Slow breathing During the early stages, calmly and deliberately breathe out through your mouth as the contraction begins. Then slowly breathe in through your nose. Sustain the same steady pattern throughout the contraction, which may last for about 45–60 seconds.

Light breathing As your contractions become more intense and frequent, you may find it easier to breathe above them. Take light, short breaths that seem to involve only the upper part of your body, and not your abdomen where the contraction is taking place. You will probably find that you use different breathing techniques at various stages of your labour.

Inhalation analgesic This is usually Entonox, or gas and oxygen – a gas that you administer yourself using a mouthpiece. You inhale deeply as the contraction starts, and carry on until the contraction peaks or you have had enough. You then put the mouthpiece aside and breathe normally. Gas works by numbing the pain centre in the brain, and can make you feel as though you're floating. You may be able to practise inhaling in an antenatal class.

Narcotics The most commonly used narcotic is pethidine, which is derived from morphine, and is given by injection in the thigh or buttock in varying dosages during the first stage of labour. It dulls the sensation of pain by acting on the nerve cells in the brain and spine. If you choose to use this, it is probably wise to ask for a small dose first to see how you are affected – you can ask for more later if you need it. It will take about 20 minutes to work. Another opioid commonly used is meptazinol (meptid).

Relief without drugs

It's important to master your chosen pain relief method, and familiarize your birth partner with the technique, before you go into labour. If any special equipment is required, make sure that it is available at home or in hospital. One method alone may not be enough – you may need a combination for complete relief.

Positions Walking around, leaning against your partner or the wall, and rocking your pelvis will probably feel much more comfortable than lying on your back in bed. There are also certain positions that you will find more comfortable than others, because these will relieve the pressure on your back (see p. 48).

Massage This is a wonderful way of getting reassurance from your partner while relieving discomfort, whether you're lying, standing, or squatting. It can be particularly relieving if you have backache during labour, which most women do (see p. 45), or if you suffer from a backache labour (see p. 70).

TENS (Trans-cutaneous Electrical Nerve Stimulation) Pain impulses conducted by nerves are blocked by an electric current, which also stimulates the production of endorphins.

A battery-powered stimulator is connected by wires to electrodes that are placed on either side of the spine. You then use a handset to regulate the amount of stimulation, and thus the pain relief that you receive.

Visualizing Creating images in your mind can be a very effective way of calming fear and reducing pain. As your contraction begins, imagine something that you find particularly soothing, for example, warm, bright sunshine. Contractions in the first stage are opening the cervix and you may find it helpful to think of the image of a bud of your favourite flower opening slowly, petal by petal. Thoughts of waves are also very comforting, the flow of the waves matching each contraction as it increases in intensity, peaks, and dies away.

Water Lying in warm water can be very relaxing and soothing because the water renders you virtually weightless and this brings relief between contractions. For these reasons, birthing pools are used by some mothers under supervision (see p. 14).

Sounds You can help to diffuse the pain and anxiety of your labour by vocalizing in the way you feel is most helpful. Sighing, moaning, groaning, and grunting are all ways of releasing tension, and you shouldn't be inhibited or worry about disturbing others.

Many women find that listening to music is very effective. Your birth partner can play different types of music depending on how you are feeling.

Hypnosis This isn't something that you should try on a whim, since you need to respond to hypnosis very easily. Women who can go into a deep trance have been able to have a forceps delivery, stitches, or Caesarean without feeling pain. A period of practice sessions is advisable, so that both you and your hypnotist are completely familiar with what you have to do during the birth.

Acupuncture You should only opt for this method if you have already found that it can relieve pain in other situations. In addition, your acupuncturist must be familiar with labour and delivery. This may not stop you feeling any pain at all, but it can reduce it, and will also help prevent nausea.

Relieving backache

Many women suffer from backache during labour, sometimes because of the baby's head pressing against the sacrum in the lower back. Massage by a birth partner can help relieve the discomfort in your lower back.

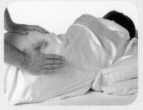

Rubbing the sacrum Using the base of your hand, rub around the lower back slowly and firmly.

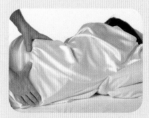

Circular pressure Press your thumbs over the sacrum and move them gently in a circle.

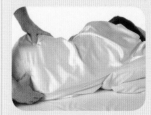

Deep pressure Press your thumbs gently but firmly into the middle of each buttock.

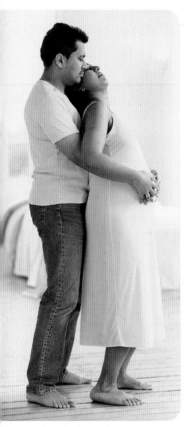

Physical support If your partner leans back against you, you can support her weight and cuddle her at the same time.

How your partner can help at the birth

The more comfortable and relaxed a mother feels during labour, the better her ability to cope with pain. She can find this security with loving support from a birth partner.

The baby's father is the natural choice, as he will probably be closely involved throughout the pregnancy and eager to share the experience of his child's birth. Most hospitals now welcome fathers, friends, or relatives to support the labouring mother.

Understanding your role

Like many partners, you may be nervous or worry about feeling squeamish, or being inadequate at offering sufficient support. You can help combat this by preparing yourself in advance. It's important that you know as much as possible so that you can effectively help the mother meet the physical and emotional demands of labour. At the antenatal classes there will be demonstrations to help you recognize the onset of labour and the effect of contractions, and you will be taught techniques to help your partner relax.

If it's going to be a hospital birth, visit the labour and delivery rooms with her and introduce yourself to her hospital attendants so you won't feel like an outsider when the time comes. If the birth is to be at home, find out what will be expected of you.

How to help during labour

You may have a very active role throughout the labour and birth, but sometimes your presence is all the mother needs. Make sure you are familiar with her birth plan and any alternative version (see p. 26). You need to be aware of her wishes in order to speak on her behalf during labour if necessary.

Use your intuition You need to judge the situation, observing your partner's moods and fitting in. She may want to stay quiet, going through her contractions alone without being touched. Alternatively, she may need a great deal of verbal or physical encouragement, or wish to be distracted by music or talking.

Provide emotional support Stay as intimate as possible, using loving words, and keep your movements slow, quiet, and steady. Always be positive: offer praise, never criticism. If she wants to hear your voice, constantly tell her how well she is doing (how far dilated), suggest how she can relax herself, tell her what other people such as the midwife are doing to help her, and what will soon happen. Also, help her to see how much she has achieved already – it's easy for her to be overwhelmed by how far she thinks she has to go. Massage and stroke her slowly if she wants you to, but if she just wants to hold your hand, you can offer encouragement simply by using facial expressions and lots of eye contact.

Combat fatigue Before labour, remind her to rest as much as possible, particularly if she seems to spend a lot of energy during the "nesting" period. If she has a long, tiring labour, try to help her relax between contractions to conserve her energy for the second stage. If she's not feeling nauseous, provide her with as much refreshment as she wants (see also p. 32). She will also probably find that having her face wiped is very soothing.

Help her cope with pain It's hard to see someone you care about in pain, but try not to reveal your anxiety because she may become discouraged. On the other hand, don't discredit her suffering. Acknowledge it positively, telling her that each contraction is bringing your baby's birth nearer, and offer different suggestions for relief. Don't let her feel embarrassed about expressing her discomfort – encourage her to be as uninhibited as possible. Try not to be upset if she becomes critical or aggressive – this often happens when the pain is very intense.

Assist with breathing You will probably have practised this during antenatal classes, but allow her to follow her own rhythm. If she seems to lose control, slowly guide her through the pattern until she can carry on alone. Be prepared to adapt – very few people follow exactly what they practised at antenatal classes.

Make her comfortable Suggest different positions, let her lean against you while you hold her, or support her with cushions. Look out for signs of tension and offer to massage or stroke her.

How the birth partner can help

A birth partner can do a lot to help during labour, not only by providing the mother with comfort and reassurance, but also by dealing with staff on her behalf. Bear in mind that although the hospital may appear daunting, the midwifery and medical team is there to support both of you. The birth partner can:

* Answer questions for the mother (if allowed to by the staff), which saves her from having her concentration disturbed.

* Support her in the positions she chooses for pain relief and/or to give birth.

* Stroke and massage her if she finds it comforting.

* Change the atmosphere (dim the lights, change the music).

* Ask people to leave if too many build up in her personal space during a home birth, and request that any students present at a hospital delivery leave if they are inhibiting the mother.

* Be the one she relies on to interact with the staff on her behalf, and to stand by her decisions regarding pain relief – whether to accept it or not, and if so, when and how much. If she does decide to ask for relief, he may encourage her to have a breathing space of about 15 minutes before it is administered, as she may find she doesn't need it after all.

First-stage positions

There are many different positions that you can adopt to ease your discomfort during the first stage. Some women prefer to stand up and move around – this helps strengthen contractions and can accelerate labour. If you do stand, try leaning forward against your partner or a wall. This will take the weight of the baby off your spine and make your contractions more efficient. As your contractions get stronger, you may instinctively choose a sitting or kneeling position, using cushions or chairs for support.

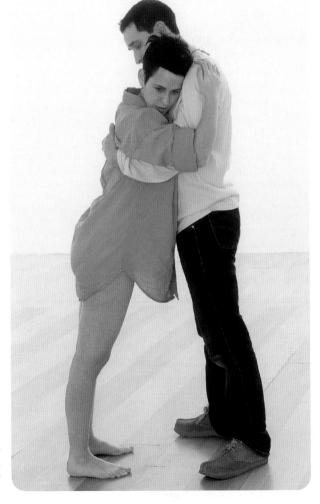

Standing Lean forward and rest against your birth partner or a wall. This position is comfortable because the weight of the baby will be taken off your spine. The contractions will be more efficient because gravity will help your baby's head to press down on the cervix. Rotate your hips. Your birth attendant will be able to help you breathe correctly. Ask your partner to massage your back as you rest against him. You may also find rocking together helps.

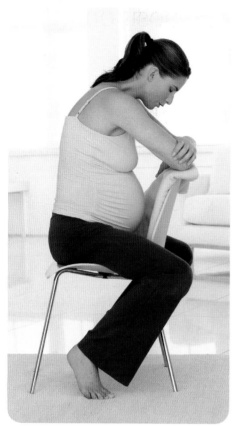

Sitting If you find it more comfortable to sit down, try leaning forward with your legs wide apart. You can sit facing the chair back, resting on a pillow or cushion during contractions. Alternatively, to keep your body supported, you may prefer to lean against your birth partner, who can also rub your back if you have low back pain. Let your shoulders drop.

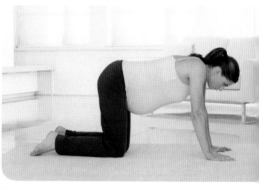

Kneeling As the contractions strengthen, instead of standing you may find it less tiring to go on your hands and knees. This will help alleviate any backache. Keep the knees wide apart, and rock your pelvis backwards and forwards during contractions. Make sure your back is straight and don't allow it to arch. Between contractions, you may need to rest your arms; you could lean forwards onto your folded arms or sit back on your heels, always making sure that your knees are wide apart (see p. 50).

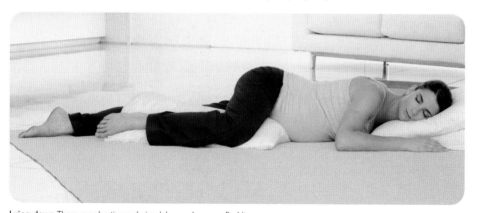

Lying down There may be times during labour when you find it more comfortable to lie down. If you wish to do so, instead of lying on your back, try lying on your side and place cushions under your head and upper thigh. Keep your legs wide apart. Relax your shoulders, and concentrate on your breathing with your eyes closed.

Transition

Transition is the last and most intense phase of the first stage. Your contractions will now last about 60–90 seconds, with intervals of only 30–90 seconds. As the contractions become stronger, you may find it difficult to relax and get comfortable. Try the two positions shown below. You may also feel a very strong urge to push, but you should not do so unless you are told that you are fully dilated. The intense pain may make you feel extremely irritable, to the point of being ill-tempered with your birth partner. Relax – this means that your baby's birth is imminent.

Resting Use this position, with your legs wide apart, to rest between contractions.

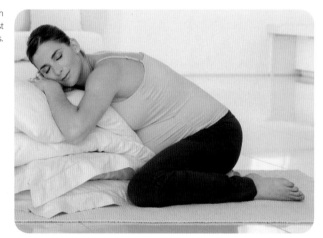

Waiting to push If your cervix is not fully dilated yet you have the urge to push, lean forward with your bottom raised and allow gravity to slow down the baby and take the pressure off your cervix.

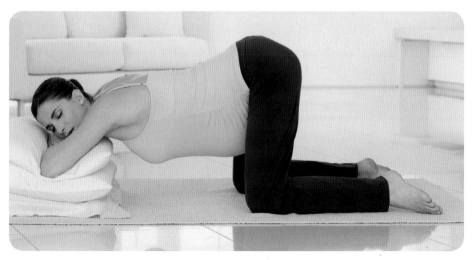

Chapter 4

Your baby is born

Your feeling of release as your baby's body slithers out after the urgency of the first and second stages of labour will be swiftly followed by a feeling of exhilaration as you greet your baby for the first time.

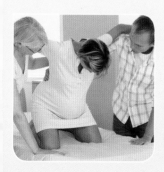
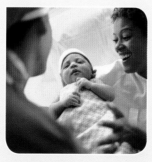
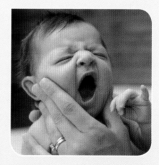

Breathing in the second stage

You will be taught breathing exercises in antenatal classes. The importance of good breathing techniques during the second stage of labour cannot be overestimated. It gives you the sensation of being in control of your own body, and during a time of stress this is very empowering.

As you begin the second stage, you may want to speed up your breathing. This is the most shallow form of breathing you should use in labour. Instead of using your chest and throat, focus on breathing only through your mouth. Breathe lightly in and out through your mouth, starting slowly and gradually quickening. Be careful not to breathe out too deeply or you will start to hyperventilate. If you feel dizzy, place your hands lightly over your nose and mouth while you are breathing.

The second stage: delivery

Delivery is the main event: it's what you've been preparing for during the last nine months. While this stage is unlikely to be painless, you can still expect to be happy and relaxed, with a birth partner of your choosing, and with equipment and surroundings that are familiar.

Contractions and pushing

The second stage is the expulsive stage when you push your baby out through the birth canal. It lasts from the full dilation of your cervix until the baby is born and, for a first baby, it usually doesn't take longer than two hours (the average is about one hour), and it may be as little as 15–20 minutes for subsequent babies. The uterine contractions are 60–90 seconds long at this time and occur at 2–4 minute intervals.

You will almost certainly feel the urge to push down, known as bearing down, which is caused by your baby's head pressing down on your pelvic floor and rectum, and is quite involuntary. Your pushing should be smooth and continuous, and all the muscular effort should be smooth and slow so that the vaginal and perineal tissues and muscles are given enough time to stretch so they will be able to accommodate your baby's head.

The most efficient position to be in when you're pushing is upright, whether you are seated on a birthing stool, standing with your arms around your partner's neck, or in a squatting position. This means that the downward muscular force of your body and the natural effect of gravity are working in unison to expel your baby. Avoid giving birth while lying on your back because in this position you're pushing your baby out uphill against the force of gravity. This requires much harder work, and therefore delivery will be slower (see p. 64). While pushing, the pelvic floor and the anal area should be fully relaxed, so make a conscious effort to let go of this part of your body. You may lose a little stool or urinate, but don't be embarrassed; it is very common and your attendants have seen it all before.

When you've finished a push, you will find two slow, deep breaths helpful, but don't relax too quickly at the end of each contraction. The baby will continue to maintain its forward progress if you relax slowly. If your second stage is considered to be prolonged, the delivery of your baby could be assisted by forceps or ventouse (see p. 74).

Normal delivery

The first sign that the baby is coming is the bulging of your anus and perineum. With each contraction, more and more of the baby's head appears at your vaginal opening, until the head doesn't slip back at all between contractions. This is known as crowning.

You will probably feel a stinging or burning sensation as the baby stretches the outlet of your vagina. As soon as you feel it, try to stop bearing down, pant, and allow the contractions of your uterus to push the baby out on its own. This may be difficult since you may still feel like pushing, but if you continue to push you increase the risk that you will tear or need an episiotomy. As you stop pushing, lean back and try to go limp. Make a conscious effort to relax the muscles of the perineal floor.

The stinging or burning sensation only lasts for a short time and is followed by a numb feeling as the baby's head stretches your vaginal tissues so that the nerves are blocked, producing a natural anaesthetic.

If the midwife suspects that you are going to tear badly, this is when she may do an episiotomy (see p. 65). She will also check that the umbilical cord is not round the baby's neck – if it is, she will gently lift it over the baby's head, make a loop through which he can be delivered or, if it is very tight, she may clamp and cut it.

When his head has been delivered, your baby will be face down, but almost immediately he will twist his head so that he is facing your left or right thigh. The midwife or other attendant will then wipe your baby's eyes, nose, and mouth, and clear any fluid from his nose.

After delivery of the head, your contractions will stop for a minute or so. When they restart, the next contraction will usually deliver one shoulder and the other shoulder will slip out. Once both shoulders are delivered, the rest of your baby will slide out quickly and easily.

Your attendants will hold him firmly because he will be slippery with blood, amniotic fluid, and possibly, *vernix caseosa*, which is the creamy substance that protects the baby's skin while he is in the womb.

What your baby does

Your baby's body goes through several twists and turns as he descends through the birth canal, all of which are intended to achieve a smooth, safe birth.

Your baby has a pliable body but a fairly firm, oval head. Both have to adapt themselves to a curved lower birth canal consisting of the lower part of the uterus inside the pelvis, the dilated cervix, and a stretched vagina. There are various adjustments that your baby makes as labour progresses.

* He will bring his chin down onto his chest as he descends through the pelvis.

* He will rotate his head.

* He will extend his head backwards, so that the back of his head touches his back as he emerges from the birth canal and vagina.

* He will make a little sideways wriggle so that his head turns to one side or the other; the shoulder of that side can then be delivered through the vagina.

* He will make another little wriggle to swing his head all the way round so that the other shoulder is delivered. (If you imagine this in quick succession, it's like a shrug of one shoulder after the other.)

* His trunk, buttocks, and legs follow his head out through the birth canal.

Giving birth

Your baby's journey down the birth canal lasts about an hour on average. You will probably feel swept along by an unbelievably strong, fundamental urge to bear down and push your baby out of the uterus, although a few women, especially if they have already had a baby, do not really experience the urge to push.

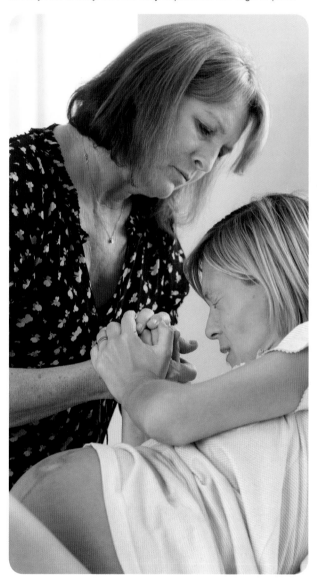

Pushing As each contraction builds until it reaches its peak, you will experience powerful urges to bear down and push your baby out. This is not something that you decide to do; it is an instinctive reaction that you will find very difficult to resist.

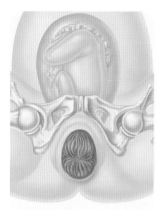

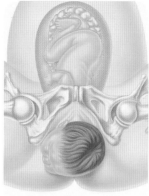

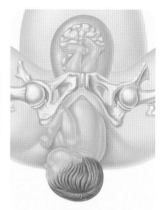

The head crowns When your baby's head does not slip back between contractions, but remains visible at the vaginal outlet, it is said to crown, and you will feel a burning or stinging sensation as your vagina stretches. Do not push at this point – allow the perineum to thin and stretch. Panting is a good way to try to control your desire to bear down. At this point, most midwives in the UK practise "HOOP" – Hands On Or Poised – so that they can easily put one hand on the baby's head if necessary, and one on the perineum.

The head emerges As her head is born, she will immediately turn it sideways. Your contractions will probably pause for a few moments at this point, and your caregivers will feel around your baby's neck to make sure that the cord is not around it. If it is, they will either lift it up over her head or make a loop through which she can be born. Her shoulders will be delivered one at a time during the next contraction or two. Everything seems to move very fast at this stage.

The baby is born As soon as her shoulders are free, the rest of her body will be born immediately. As she slithers out of your vagina, she will usually be followed by a great gush of amniotic fluid. Your caregivers will hold her carefully as she will be slippery with blood and the thick, greasy substance known as *vernix caseosa*. She may be breathing and crying already.

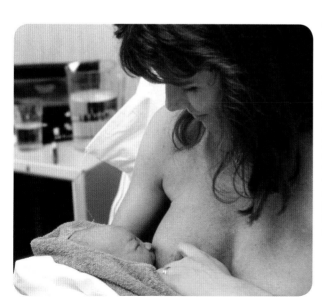

The first cuddle Your caregivers will often place your baby immediately onto your tummy and then cover her in a blanket to keep her warm. Or they may wipe her face and clear her air passages first, then give her to you to hold in the few minutes after her birth. She may start to suckle spontaneously, but if she doesn't, you could bring her to your breast and offer the nipple to her cheek, which will encourage her to turn and take it. Don't be upset if she does not seem interested just yet – she is probably just getting used to the idea. Now you and your partner can enjoy a cuddle with your new baby.

How the birth partner can help

By the second stage of labour, the birth partner's role in providing loving support for the mother will be well-established. She has now passed through the most painful phase and has reached the climactic stage of delivery.

Second stage jobs

Many of the jobs you performed during the first stage – making her comfortable, supporting different positions, providing refreshment, and giving moral support – may also be needed at this stage. However, this is when you will also have to encourage her to push. All this will make the mother's work very much easier and help her feel emotionally secure and relaxed.

If you are in hospital and are suddenly asked to leave the delivery room, do so without question. There may be a medical emergency and staff will have to move quickly. You cannot guarantee that you will not be in the way, so leave the delivery room but stay nearby.

Helping with the delivery position Your partner will probably know by now which position she finds the most comfortable. You can offer valuable support to help her through the pushing

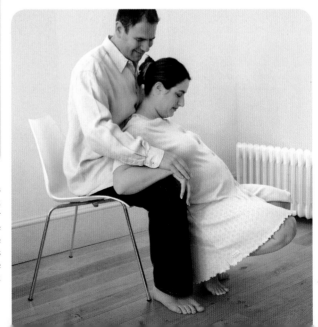

Supported squat If your partner's happy for you to be close to her, she can lean back against you for support. You will be able to guide her through the contractions. The closeness of your body next to hers may help make her feel more relaxed during the delivery.

stage, but don't hesitate to ask the midwife for advice if you're not certain what you have to do. If your partner doesn't want to be held, you can offer suggestions for other positions that she may find comfortable, and place pillows or cushions behind her for support. If your partner is happy sitting in bed or on the floor, suggest that she try the knee-chest position, which many women find comfortable during the second stage. She should drop her chin on to her chest while holding on to her knees.

Helping her with breathing and pushing To help her through these last few contractions, tap out a rhythm for the different kinds of breathing, using words like breathe, breathe, pant, pant, blow. As she's pushing, gently remind her to relax her pelvic floor.

At the peak of contractions, suggest that she take two or three deep breaths and push as hard as she can. She should push in a steady way, and you can remind her that each push brings the birth of your baby nearer.

Encouraging her to relax Make sure she relaxes fully between contractions because she needs to conserve her strength for pushing her baby through the birth canal. Massage her back (see pp. 44–45) if she has backache or just needs reassurance. If she is hot, mop her brow or spray her face with water.

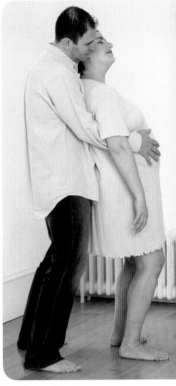

Standing position If your partner wants to deliver the baby standing up, you can help support her by standing behind her and taking her weight on your arms. In this position, her pelvis will be completely open and she'll be able to take full advantage of gravity. She should hold her legs wide apart.

Standing by Once the baby's head has crowned, you may then have a more passive role and become an observer. The midwife will guide your partner through this pushing stage. Don't be disappointed if the mother doesn't communicate with you during this part of the birth and seems to rely more on the midwife. She will now be fully preoccupied and involved, and may not notice you for some time.

Showing her the baby When the baby's head is emerging, offer to hold a mirror nearby so that she can see his head crowning and then his whole body slithering out. Encourage her to reach down and touch her baby's head as he is born.

Loving reception With the assistance of the midwife, you may be able to "catch" your baby as his body emerges. After you have greeted him for the first time, place him on your partner's stomach. You can then cuddle them both to help to keep them warm and to let them know that you're there and that you love them.

What the placenta looks like

Many first-time mothers are very interested in seeing their baby's placenta.

The placenta measures about 20–25 centimetres (8–10 inches) in diameter and weighs about 0.5 kilograms (1 pound). It is disc-shaped and its surfaces are very different in appearance.

The fetal side was continuous with the wall of your uterus and covered by membranes. It is flat and smooth, and is blue-grey in colour with blood vessels radiating out from the umbilical cord. The maternal side is dark red and looks like several pieces of raw liver joined together.

The third stage

Once your baby has been born, your uterus will rest for about 15 minutes. It will then start to contract again in order to expel the placenta. This is called the third stage of labour and it is comparatively painless – you will probably hardly notice it.

The final stage

During this stage of labour the placenta becomes detached from the uterine wall and is delivered by expulsion down the birth canal. The large blood vessels, which are about the thickness of a pencil and which run to and from the placenta, are simply torn across. However, bleeding is rare because the muscle fibres of the uterus are arranged in a criss-cross fashion, which means that when the uterus contracts, the muscles tighten around the blood vessels and prevent them from bleeding.

This is why it is absolutely essential that the uterus contracts down into a hard ball once the placenta has been expelled. The uterus can be kept tightly contracted by massaging it intermittently for an hour or so afterwards. Normally, the third stage lasts up to an hour, but with active management (see p. 59) this can be much shorter.

The placenta is delivered

Traditionally, no attempt is made to deliver the placenta until there are clear signs that it is separating from the uterine wall and moving downwards into the vagina. The signs that your attendants will look for are the resumption of contractions a few minutes after the birth of your baby and a desire to bear down on your part, which indicates that the placenta has separated from the uterine wall and is pressing down on your pelvic floor.

Delivery When these signs occur, delivery of the placenta is encouraged by the birth attendant pulling gently on the cord and at the same time pressing above the rim of the pelvis to control descent. The placenta is delivered, followed by the membranes.

Many women want to see the placenta – this is very understandable because this amazing organ has been the life-support system for your baby during the nine months of your pregnancy.

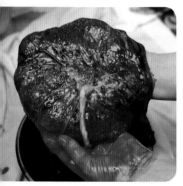

The placenta The side of the placenta that was facing towards your baby is flat and smooth. Note the umbilical cord emerging from its centre and the prominent blood vessels.

After delivery Once the placenta is delivered, your midwife will carefully examine it to make sure that it is complete and that none of it has been left behind. If any of the placenta has been retained by the uterus it can be a cause of haemorrhage later on, so it should be removed as soon as the diagnosis is made. The membranes should be a complete bag except for the hole through which the fetus has passed. The cut end of the cord is examined to check that the umbilical blood vessels are normal. After the placenta is delivered, the entire vulval outlet will be examined carefully for tears, and anything other than a tiny one must be stitched immediately.

Management of the third stage

Using a hormonal drug known as ergometrine, doctors and midwives now actively manage the third stage of labour. Given ergometrine at the time of birth, or immediately after, the number of cases of excessive bleeding, defined as loss of more than 500 millilitres of blood (1 pint), is reduced.

Ergometrine causes prolonged contraction of the uterus without a period of relaxation, and while the uterus is contracted there is not likely to be any bleeding. The placenta will separate very quickly from the uterine wall once the uterus starts to contract, thereby shortening the third stage of labour.

Syntometrine Nowadays, most attendants use a combination of ergometrine and syntocinon known as syntometrine. This is because ergometrine on its own is rather slow to start to work and can cause nausea, so using it with syntocinon, which acts quickly to stimulate uterine contractions, gives a better result.

Syntometrine is given by intramuscular injection into your thigh just when the head is crowning or with delivery of the first shoulder, and is used automatically in the majority of hospital births to reduce the risk of postpartum haemorrhage (see column, right). The hormone oxytocin is also naturally produced by your body in response to seeing and touching your baby, and by putting her to your breast. It does the same job as the injection, but is less reliable.

How you'll feel

You may find yourself shivering with cold after the placenta is delivered. This shivering, which produces body heat by the rapid contraction and relaxation of the muscles, usually passes in about half an hour.

Postpartum haemorrhage

This is rare, largely because the uterus has a self-protecting device to stop it from bleeding.

Once the uterus is completely empty, it contracts down to about the size of a tennis ball. The contraction of the uterine muscles nips the uterine arteries so that they cannot bleed. Under normal circumstances, therefore, little bleeding occurs after the delivery. What little bleeding there is appears as the lochia – the usual postpartum vaginal discharge (see p. 84).

A uterus in which remnants of the placenta are retained may bleed, and this bleeding is called postpartum haemorrhage. It is usually diagnosed by examining the placenta and finding that a portion is missing. The mother may be given an anaesthetic and the placenta is gently scraped away from inside the uterus.

If bleeding occurs more than 24 hours after delivery, the lochia may become bright red again. This can occur as a result of being too energetic. Consult your doctor, who will probably advise you to rest for several days. If the bleeding recurs or becomes heavy, this can be a sign of infection or of the retention of a small piece of placenta. Contact your doctor immediately. If you pass large clots of blood, call an ambulance and ask to be taken to the nearest emergency unit.

Your new baby

When your baby has been delivered, before the cord is cut and various checks have been carried out (see p. 62), he will be handed to you. Holding your baby soon after birth will help you to establish a strong emotional bond with him. Your baby will start to learn about you by hearing your voice, smelling and feeling your skin, and being cuddled and suckled.

A newborn baby's tiny, vulnerable body and complete dependence will arouse many new emotions. Research has shown that parents who are given unrestricted contact with their babies immediately after delivery tend to be more sympathetic to their children's needs later than parents whose babies are taken away at birth. A lack of initial contact can make some mothers feel alienated from their babies, and so, less attentive.

What your baby looks like

What is considered normal for the weight and length of a newborn varies within a range. Average weights are between 2.5 and 4.5 kilograms (5lb 8oz–9lb 12oz), and average lengths between 48 and 51 centimetres (19–20 inches).

Head This is still large in comparison with the rest of his body. It usually has a pointed shape because it has been moulded as it came through the birth canal. Moulding is caused by the skull bones overriding each other. Sometimes this pressure also causes swelling on one or both sides of the head. This swelling leaves the brain unaffected and subsides in a few weeks.

There may be slight bruising around the scalp if your baby was delivered by forceps or ventouse. You will feel a soft spot on the top, called the anterior fontanelle, where the skull bones have not yet joined together – this won't close up until your baby is 18 months old.

Skin Some babies are born completely covered in a greasy, white substance called *vernix caseosa*, others have it only on their face and hands. Vernix eases the baby's delivery and offers protection against minor skin infections. In some hospitals it is cleaned off immediately, in others it is left to rub off the skin naturally within two or three days.

You may notice downy hair, known as lanugo, on his body; it covered your baby's body while he was in your uterus. Some babies only have it on the head, while on others it covers the shoulders. Both are quite normal and the hair usually rubs off in a couple of weeks. More permanent hair will appear later.

Hands and feet These are always slightly more bluish than the rest of his body because his circulation hasn't yet stabilized. There may be dry patches with peeling skin, which will disappear in a few days. His fingernails may be long and sharp; you can gently nibble off the tips if he's getting scratched, but don't cut them.

Umbilicus The clamped umbilical cord doesn't separate from the navel until about 10 days after birth. Some babies have umbilical hernias (small swellings near the navel) but these usually clear up within a year.

Breasts In both boy and girl babies, the breasts may be slightly enlarged and leak a little milk, owing to pregnancy hormones; this is normal and will stop in a few days.

Your newborn

Your baby's legs may look bowed because he has been curled up in your uterus

Your baby's skin colour will change frequently and look blotchy

A beating pulse may be seen under the fontanelle. It should never be pressed hard

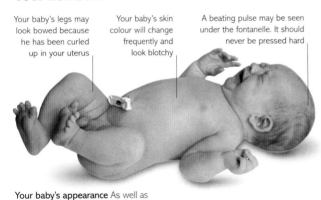

Your baby's appearance As well as puffy eyelids and a blotched and spotty skin surface, he will have enlarged genitals.

Your baby's birthmarks

A group of small blood vessels under the surface of the skin may appear as a blemish on your baby's body, but won't usually need any treatment.

Stork bites These are mild pink patches; they are very common and usually appear on the nose, eyelids, and neck. They take about a year to fade.

Strawberry birthmarks These first appear as tiny red dots and may increase in size up to the end of the first year. They almost always disappear by the age of five.

Mongolian spots These are blue and are found on the lower backs of babies with dark skin tones. The spots look like bruises, but they are harmless and will fade away.

Port wine stains These are large, flat, red or purple marks on the baby's skin. They are often found on the face and neck. They are permanent, so if you are worried consult your doctor.

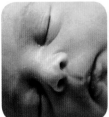

Puffy eyelids

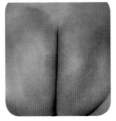

Blotchy skin tone

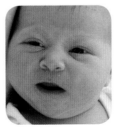

Spotty skin

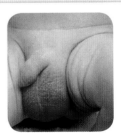

Enlarged genitals

The Apgar score

Within a minute of birth, five simple tests are carried out to see whether your baby is fit and healthy. These are scored on the Apgar scale (named after Dr Virginia Apgar, who devised it). The score includes the following:

Pulse/heart rate This measures the strength and regularity of the heartbeat. 100 beats per minute scores 2, below 100 scores 1, no pulse scores 0.

Breathing This reveals the maturity and health of the baby's lungs. Regular breathing scores 2, irregular 1, none 0.

Movements An indication of the baby's muscle tone. Active movements score 2, some movements 1, limp scores 0.

Skin colour This shows how well the lungs are working to oxygenate the blood. Pink skin scores 2, bluish extremities 1, totally blue skin scores 0.

Reflexes Crying and grimacing reveal that the baby responds to stimuli. Crying scores 2, whimpering 1, silence 0.

Most babies score between 7 and 10. A second test is done five minutes later.

Your baby will be examined by the doctor or midwife to make sure her facial features and body proportions are normal. They will also check her fingers and toes, and her back for signs of spina bifida.

Just after delivery

Once your baby is delivered, all of the attention will be given to her, not to you, and rightly so. She may cry first when delivered and will be crying lustily a few seconds after birth. She will probably be a bluish-white colour at first and may be covered with *vernix caseosa* (see p. 60).

Cutting the cord The first procedure is the clamping of the cord. It is now generally believed that the baby benefits from the return of placental blood through the umbilical cord, and that the cord should not be clamped until it stops pulsating. Blood can flow from the placenta to the baby only if the baby is at a lower level than the uterus. At the appropriate time, two clamps are applied to the cord, one a short distance from the navel, the other about 2 centimetres (1 inch) away from the first. These clamps prevent the cord from bleeding, the one closest to the baby being the most important. The cord is then cut between the clamps. It may have been clamped and cut during delivery if it was looped tightly around the baby's neck.

Her general condition The midwife will check your baby's general condition. She will remove any remaining fluid in the baby's mouth, nose, or air passages by sucking it out with a plastic tube. If the baby doesn't start breathing immediately, the midwife will give her oxygen.

Welcoming your baby

Once the wellbeing of your baby is established, by all means ask the midwifery and medical staff to leave if you wish to be alone with your partner and your baby. You can both relax after your hard work and enjoy this amazing new experience. It's a good idea to put your baby to the breast immediately, even if your baby isn't hungry.

Spend these initial few minutes concentrating on your baby, getting to know her, learning to recognize her face, and cooing at her so that she can hear the sound of your voice. You should hold her about 20–25 centimetres (8–10 inches) away from you because at this distance she can make out your face quite clearly. Smile and talk gently in a sing-song voice because newborn babies are attuned to high vocal pitches.

Chapter 5

Special circumstances

Most labours are quite straightforward, but some are complicated and require special techniques. But since each birth is unique and special for every woman, it will still be your labour – and entirely memorable.

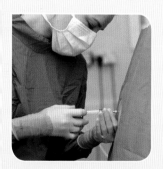

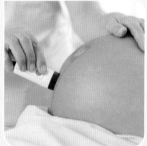

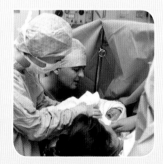

Disadvantages of lying down

Although fetal monitoring (see p. 67) may confine you to bed, lying on your back for delivery can have many disadvantages.

* You have to work harder pushing the baby uphill.

* Pain may be greater in this position than in a vertical one.

* The tissues of the birth canal may be slow to open which may prolong labour.

* There may be a greater need for an episiotomy and an increased chance of an assisted delivery.

* It inhibits spontaneous delivery of the placenta.

* There is a greater possibility of lower back strain.

Speeding up delivery

What is considered to be the normal length of labour varies from hospital to hospital. If medical staff attending to you feel that your labour needs to be sped up, they may use the following procedures:

* Rupturing the membranes or setting up a syntocinon drip

* Use of episiotomy (see p. 65) and assisted delivery

The modern way

Certain procedures historically associated with childbirth are being re-evaluated. Some have been found to be unnecessary, others unjustified. However, most of today's obstetricians believe that they can guarantee that childbirth is a safer and happier experience for both mother and baby with the help of modern technology.

By drawing your attention to the arguments concerning some standard medical practices, this chapter will help you to question them assertively with your medical and midwifery attendants. More often than not, your wishes will be complied with, especially if you have written a birth plan in advance (see p.26), but occasionally you will be told that to continue with a particular option could put you or your baby at serious risk – for instance, if your baby is showing signs of distress and you insist on continuing with a totally natural childbirth. Be prepared to adapt your ideas according to what is best for you and your baby.

Shaving Nowadays, shaving is unnecessary unless you are having a Caesarean section. Any chance of infection can be eliminated by simply spraying the vulva with an antiseptic and wiping with gauze.

Nil by mouth Many modern obstetric units have abandoned the old custom of nil by mouth but some hospitals may still practise it. There is no medical or scientific rationale for starving a woman during labour. In fact, quite the opposite: the hard work of labour uses up much energy, and causes sweating, and a woman must replace the fluids and energy that she has lost.

In times past, Caesarean sections were performed under general anaesthetic, which could not be given to a woman who had eaten recently, in case she vomited and choked. Nowadays, however, most Caesareans are carried out under an epidural, which has no such risks. In any case, there is no reason why every woman should still suffer simply because a small number may need surgical intervention.

Moving to a delivery room In some hospitals a woman still has to undergo the physical and emotional upheaval of leaving the room where she started labour in order to have her baby in a delivery room. Ideally, labour should proceed smoothly in peaceful surroundings, and as long as a room is equipped with good lighting, oxygen in some form, and a suction apparatus to clear out the baby's air passages if necessary, I can see no reason why a woman in normal labour should be forced to move to a delivery room. Many progressive hospitals now have more congenial all-in-one labour and birthing rooms, and if possible, you should choose a hospital with these.

Induction Starting off labour artificially is not a new idea, but it only became an easy procedure in the latter half of the 20th century. Labour is usually induced for medical reasons, such as pre-eclampsia, high blood pressure, or post-maturity, when induction can save the lives of mothers and babies (see pp. 68–69). An induced labour may involve the use of a syntocinon drip, which will restrict your movements. Such a labour can be shorter and sharper and probably will increase your need for heavy-duty painkillers.

Amniotomy This is when the membranes (the bag of waters surrounding the baby) are artificially ruptured (see p. 69). It may be carried out in a high-tech birth, and if so, is usually done early in labour for three reasons: the first is so that electronic fetal monitoring equipment can be set in place, the second is to check if the amniotic fluid contains meconium (this is the baby's first bowel movement and its presence may indicate fetal distress), and the third is that once the membranes are ruptured, the baby's head can press down hard on the cervix, helping the dilation of the cervix and speeding up the first stage. Amniotomy can only be done if the cervix is already partially dilated.

Episiotomy This is a surgical cut to enlarge the vaginal outlet at delivery (see column, right), and is the most commonly performed operation in the West. Episiotomies are employed in order to avoid tears, which have ragged edges and are difficult to stitch together. They can also take longer to heal. Tears can be avoided if a woman is encouraged to stop pushing while the head is being born, allowing her uterus to ease out the head gradually rather than quickly. When the head delivers too fast, an episiotomy may be done because the perineum is thought to be under stress. If you wish to avoid an episiotomy, have it noted that you don't want one unless absolutely necessary.

The unkindest cut?

An episiotomy is an incision that helps deliver a baby's head; it isn't always needed if the head is delivered slowly.

If you have already had an epidural for your labour, you will probably not need any further anaesthetic, unless it has worn off, in which case it may be topped up.

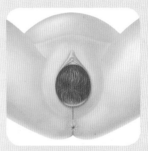

The mid-line cut This is performed by cutting straight down into the perineum, between the vagina and anus.

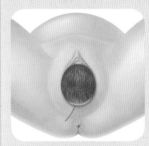

The medio-lateral cut This is angled down and away from the vagina and perineum into the muscle. A local anaesthetic in your perineum is usually necessary beforehand.

The older mother

Towards the end of pregnancy, obstetricians are always on the lookout for signs of placental insufficiency as the baby outgrows the food supply. Older mothers especially come in for careful scrutiny.

The timing of induction of labour should be one of the questions you should ask if the subject doesn't come up for discussion. Of course, induction is not always necessary. A mother who reaches her estimated date of delivery, given that she and her baby are perfectly normal, should be allowed to go into spontaneous labour. I would strongly advocate, however, that once the EDD has been passed, you co-operate with the frequent monitoring of your condition and that of the baby, and if there is any sign of fetal distress, agree to have medical intervention.

Are you overdue?

Only about five per cent of all babies arrive on the date that they are expected. The estimated date of delivery (EDD) is only a statistical average, and studies have shown that as many as 40 per cent of babies are born more than a week after their EDD.

Being overdue

One of the main difficulties in deciding whether a baby is actually overdue or not is that the precise date of conception in any particular pregnancy is unknown. Even if you have a regular menstrual cycle of 28 days (the standard on which the EDD chart is based), the date of ovulation is only known approximately. Apart from this uncertainty about the date of ovulation, every baby is different and therefore it is unrealistic to expect all babies to mature in precisely the same number of days. Moreover, since labour is initiated by your baby producing certain hormones as he reaches full maturity, the actual date of delivery can vary fairly widely, even in "textbook" pregnancies.

However, doctors do become concerned if a pregnancy continues much beyond the estimated date of delivery. This is because post-maturity and possible placental insufficiency pose risks to the health of the baby.

Most units suggest that the membranes are "swept" at approximately 41 weeks and induction is arranged for between the 41st and 42nd weeks. A membrane sweep involves an internal examination by your midwife or doctor to stimulate natural prostaglandin release (see p. 68) and hopefully start labour off naturally.

Pelvic disproportion Labour may be delayed if your baby's head is too big to pass through your pelvis. This disproportion may prevent the baby's head from becoming engaged. If this is the case, for the safety of the baby, it may be suggested that he be delivered by Caesarean section.

Post-maturity

An overdue baby faces the danger of being post-mature. A post-mature baby will have lost fat from all over his body, particularly his tummy. Consequently, his skin will look red and wrinkled as if it doesn't fit him, and it may have begun to peel. Very few babies are actually post-mature, but because post-maturity depends not only on the baby, but also on the placenta, it is difficult to predict which babies will be at risk.

Risks These include a longer and more difficult labour, because the post-mature baby tends to be bigger and the bones in his skull tend to be harder (which means that his descent through the birth canal is likely to be more traumatic both for him and for you). There is also an increased risk of stillbirth (the risk doubles by the 43rd week and triples by the 44th week). A further risk is that a uterus that is slow to start labour may also be relatively inefficient during labour.

Monitoring the overdue baby

Babies past their EDD are monitored closely, and there are a number of different ways of doing this.

Fetal movement recording The most accurate sign
that all is well with your baby is if you can detect regular fetal movements. Since all babies are different, the amount of activity that is normal for each individual pregnancy varies. You are the best judge of whether your unborn baby is acting normally, and you can monitor his activity by making a note of how many kicks you feel in a day.

Electronic fetal monitoring This may be used to check the
baby's heartbeat by providing a continuous sound and paper recording. If his heartbeat is satisfactory, it is usually considered unnecessary to perform other tests.

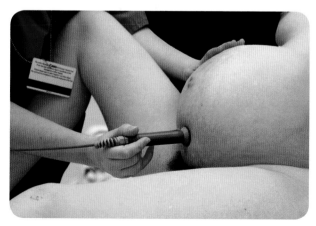

Hand-held monitor A hand-held external monitor is used for short periods of routine monitoring. This battery-operated Doppler ultrasound device allows midwives to assess the fetus' heartbeat throughout labour.

Reasons for induction

Anything that makes the uterine environment unhealthy for the baby is a reason for induction. Your labour is likely to be induced if:

✳ You suffer from hypertension, pre-eclampsia, heart disease, diabetes, or antepartum bleeding.

✳ Your carers judge that the placenta is weakening (so that the baby is in danger of not getting enough nutrients and oxygen from the placenta).

✳ Your pregnancy is prolonged beyond 42 weeks.

✳ Your waters have broken and there are no signs of labour starting naturally.

Induction of labour

Traditionally, induction of labour was undertaken by artificially rupturing the membranes and giving oxytocin to stimulate uterine contractions. The same techniques are used to accelerate labour if the contractions are weak and progress is slow. Nowadays, more gentle techniques are used by means of prostaglandin pessaries or gel.

Most inductions are elective, which means they are not emergency procedures and your baby is not in jeopardy. Your partner will be able to be with you at all times. If you're in any doubt about why your doctor is suggesting induction of labour, ask for a detailed explanation – this should cover the range of alternatives.

The history of induction

Forty years ago when the relevant drugs first became available, induction of labour was frequently used for hospital or social convenience. Occasionally, a woman might ask to be induced so that the birth could fall on her husband's birthday, or so that the child would be the right age for the school year! Such reasons are no longer accepted as valid.

When induction first became fashionable, today's technological back-up, such as ultrasound scanning, was not available for doctors to establish fetal maturity, and so babies could be born too early and suffer respiratory problems. The number of Caesarean sections also rose. Nowadays, fewer than 1 in 5 labours are induced.

As only five per cent of babies actually come on the expected due date, it can be hard for some doctors – and quite a lot of mothers – to remain philosophical when that magic date passes. There may also be concern that the placenta may be becoming inadequate to support the baby.

How induction is done

Whether induction is elective or an emergency procedure, most obstetric units will normally use a combination of three different methods to induce labour.

Prostaglandin pessaries One of the more modern methods of induction is by the use of prostaglandin pessaries or gel, which soften the cervix, causing the woman to go into labour. Pessaries are inserted into the vagina during the evening and

you may be lucky enough to be in labour by morning. This
is a satisfactory method of induction because you can move
freely around the ward.

Artificial rupture of the membranes (ARM) Also known
as amniotomy, this method of induction, often accompanied
by a syntocinon drip (see below), involves an instrument not
unlike a crochet hook being inserted into the uterus to make
an opening in the membrane so that the waters escape. This
is a painless procedure because the amniotic membranes are
entirely insensitive. Labour usually reaches full intensity quickly
after ARM because the baby's head is no longer cushioned, and
presses down hard against the cervix, encouraging the uterus
to contract and the cervix to dilate. Amniotomy is occasionally
used to speed up the first part of labour. It is not just a method
of induction – it can also be performed if an electrode needs
to be attached to the baby's scalp to monitor its heartbeat (see
p. 41). It is also performed if the baby's heart rate goes down
because of distress. In this case, traces of meconium, the baby's
first bowel movement, may be seen in the amniotic fluid.

Syntocinon-induced labour Labour is stimulated by a
natural hormone called oxytocin, produced in the posterior
pituitary gland in the brain. A synthetic form of oxytocin,
called syntocinon, is used to induce labour.

Syntocinon is given in a drip, so ask for it to be inserted
in the arm you use least and check if you can have a long tube
connecting you to the drip. This will give you more room to move
around, even if just on the bed. Contractions brought on by a
hormone drip are often stronger, longer, and more painful than
normal, with shorter periods of rest between them, increasing
the need for painkilling drugs. As the blood supply to the
uterus is temporarily shut off during each strong contraction,
it's possible that this may be detrimental to the fetus.

Expectations of induced labour

If properly handled, induced labour need not be more painful or
difficult than natural labour. If syntocinon is used, your doctor
or midwife should be able to get you to the stage where you
have a normal labour. If you prefer a completely natural childbirth,
you can still breathe through the contractions and push the baby
out at your own pace. If labour does become too painful, which
it may, you can request some form of pain relief (see pp. 42–43).

The way your baby is positioned can affect your labour and delivery. The usual presentation is head down with the baby's spine outwards (top), but your baby's spine can face inwards (middle), or she can be buttocks down (breech).

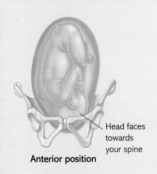

Head faces towards your spine

Anterior position

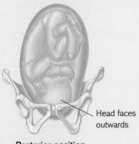

Head faces outwards

Posterior position

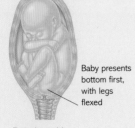

Baby presents bottom first, with legs flexed

Breech position

Special types of labour

Most labours are quite straightforward, but occasionally a complication may arise that necessitates the use of special treatment. With vigilant antenatal care, potential problems should be anticipated and assistance given, but sometimes the first stage of labour may be well underway before the problem is identified.

Backache labour

Occasionally, the discomfort of uterine contractions will be experienced primarily as low back pain. This is usually due to the stretching of the cervix as it dilates.

It may also occur if your baby lies in the posterior position (see column, left) with the back of his head up against your spine (1 in 10 babies lie in this position, so it is not abnormal).

In the posterior position, your baby's neck may not be properly flexed and a larger proportion than normal of the head presents, which may prolong labour. Usually, the baby will rotate 180 degrees into the anterior position and labour will proceed smoothly. If, as occasionally happens, the baby fails to rotate to the anterior position, this is no cause for alarm, although your doctor may need to assist with the delivery.

This type of labour may start slowly and be protracted, so it can be very tiring. There are various ways in which you and your birth partner can relieve your backache:

Massage This is the most effective way of relieving backache (see p. 44). However, if you find that being touched by someone else is irritating during your contractions, particularly during transition, you may prefer to use your own knuckles by placing a hand underneath each buttock.

Change in position When you are lying flat on your back, your baby is pressing down hardest on your spine and its nerves. Try to stay upright and walk around as much as possible. You can also relieve the pressure of your baby on your spine by sitting tailor-fashion, by leaning forward, or by rocking your pelvis. If you feel more comfortable lying down, lie on the side that your baby is facing (ask your midwife about this).

Application of heat In the early stages, a hot shower, particularly if directed on to your back, may provide some relief. You may also find it helpful if, during or between contractions, your birth partner places a heated pad against the lower part of your back.

Prolonged labour

Labour is said to be prolonged when strong uterine contractions fail to bring about the delivery. This may be due to the inability of the cervix to dilate or failure of the baby to descend through the birth canal. Doctors keep a very careful eye on the length of each stage of labour. When labour appears to be progressing more slowly than normal, your obstetrician may suspect obstruction and take an early decision to intervene – with an assisted delivery or a Caesarean section.

No woman is allowed to go on with a difficult birth for much over the accepted time (see p. 39) as this may lead to maternal exhaustion and fetal distress. Obstruction can be more quickly detected in a mother who has had several children. However, your doctor or midwife will be monitoring your general condition throughout labour, and he or she will be alerted to possible obstruction if your condition appears to deteriorate.

With a very long labour, if you are foregoing food and rest, you might eventually become too tired or distressed to push adequately. Your doctor and midwife will try to avoid this happening.

Failure to dilate When contractions are weak and infrequent, with the cervix dilating slowly, the uterus may be failing to contract forcefully enough. One way in which your doctor and midwife can tell exactly how your labour is progressing is by plotting a partogram or graph. If the failure of the uterus to contract efficiently is the only reason for the lack of progress, your doctor may begin special procedures to speed up the thinning and dilation of the cervix. The membranes may be artificially ruptured and then, if necessary, syntocinon may be administered intravenously with a drip or a pump. The dosage will be increased until strong contractions are occurring about every three minutes. Close attention is paid to make sure there is no excessive increase in the strength or frequency of contractions.

Causes of fetal obstruction

Certain fetal conditions may cause you to have an obstructed labour. Fortunately, these problems can usually be detected early on, so that your medical team can take action to help. They usually occur when:

∗ Your baby is too large.

∗ Your baby is lying in a transverse or oblique position.

∗ Your baby is in a breech, face, or brow presentation.

∗ Your baby is lying in the posterior position.

∗ Your twin babies are entwined.

∗ Your baby has a congenital abnormality, such as hydrocephalus.

Causes of obstruction

If your labour is not progressing normally, there may be reasons why your pelvis or uterus is obstructing the descent of your baby.

✳ Deformity or disproportion of the bony pelvis.

✳ Pelvic masses, such as fibroids or an ovarian cyst.

✳ Abnormalities of the uterus, cervix, or vagina.

✳ A contraction ring of the uterus, which is when the uterus pulls in excessively and a band of tight muscles occurs. This can stop contractions passing all the way down and may result in constriction of the uterus or cervix. Fortunately, it is very rare unless the uterus has been overstimulated by syntocinon or prostaglandin, such as during induction (see p. 68). In this instance, a Caesarean section is almost always required.

Failure to descend One other reason for an obstructed labour is disproportion. Disproportion results if the size of your baby's head and the size of your pelvis fail to match up. If your pelvis is too small relative to your baby's head, disproportion results. It is easy to understand how your baby might not descend in such circumstances.

If you're a first-time mother and your baby is still high and non-engaged during the last few weeks of your pregnancy, your doctor may suspect disproportion. This will also be taken into account if the baby's head remains high during labour, despite strong contractions.

If the disproportion is quite slight, there are no other irregularities, and the baby's head is believed to be descending, your doctor may let you have a trial of labour, which is where you start labour normally, but if progress is slow, you will not be allowed to continue (remember that it is your uterus on trial, not you). Once the head has entered the pelvic cavity, a vaginal delivery usually follows. If the disproportion is major, doctors will perform a Caesarean section.

Premature labour

A premature labour is one that occurs at less than 37 weeks of gestation. In about 40 per cent of cases the cause is a mystery. It is, however, known to occur in the following instances: premature rupture of the membranes, multiple pregnancy, pre-eclampsia, cervical incompetence, and uterine abnormalities. Overwork, stress, and some maternal diseases, such as anaemia or malnutrition, may also have an effect.

Knowing whether you've actually gone into premature labour is almost as difficult for your doctors and midwives as it is for you (see p. 73). As a general rule, a premature labour begins without any warning; the first sign may be rupture of the membranes, the beginning of uterine contractions, or some vaginal bleeding. There is no stopping labour if your membranes have ruptured and labour has begun, but if the membranes are intact, certain measures can be taken.

What you can do If your membranes have ruptured but labour hasn't started within 48 hours, you must contact your doctor or midwife. Rest if you are advised to stay at home, or go into hospital if asked to do so. Do not have sexual intercourse. Apart from these precautions, it is inadvisable to try to suppress labour once the membranes have ruptured spontaneously, as there is a risk of infection occuring. In fact, if contractions do not begin on their own within a day or so, syntocinon is usually given in order to encourage them to start.

What can be done by the hospital If you are experiencing premature contractions but your waters have not broken, the main aim of hospitalization is to give you treatment that may delay or suppress labour so that your child can remain in your uterus for as long as possible, thereby continuing to be nourished by you. This is because a preterm baby has an increased risk of developing respiratory distress syndrome, and the shorter the gestation period, the greater the risk.

If your pregnancy is less than 34 weeks gestation or your baby weighs less than 1.5 kilograms (3 pounds), and your cervix is less than 5 centimetres (2 inches) dilated with the membranes still intact, the hospital can offer you bed-rest to improve uterine blood supply, and more rarely, drugs to suppress labour. Additionally, in cases of premature rupture of the membranes, your doctor will check for evidence of infection and monitor your baby's condition.

All of the drugs cause some side-effects, and for that reason, only certain cases of premature labour are eligible to receive them. The main criteria for drug treatment are that you are healthy; you have no heart disease, diabetes, high blood pressure, or an abnormally placed placenta; and that there is no evidence of a congenital defect.

If you are very anxious, a mild sedative may be given to you, but morphine and pethidine should not be administered unless your pain is extremely severe. These drugs may make your uterine muscles more irritable rather than calming them down.

Managing labour As a general rule, premature labour tends to be shorter and easier than full-term, mainly because the baby's head is smaller and softer. However, an episiotomy is usually given to protect the baby's head from pressure changes within the birth canal. Your medical team will take special care to avoid hypoxia (a lack of oxygen to the tissues) throughout your labour and delivery. It may be necessary to deliver some premature babies by Caesarean section, particularly if there is fetal distress. Your baby should have vitamin K after delivery to help prevent bleeding into the brain, a particular problem with premature babies.

Premature labour?

Here are some useful pointers for diagnosing whether or not you have gone into premature labour:

* You are less than 37 weeks into your pregnancy.

* You have experienced contractions for at least an hour.

* Contractions occur every 5–10 minutes.

* Contractions last for 30 seconds and persist over the period of an hour.

* A vaginal examination by your doctor or midwife shows that your cervix is more than 2 centimetres (1 inch) dilated and the cervix is effacing.

By following these criteria, two-thirds of all patients who think they are in premature labour will actually be found not to be in real labour, and no treatment will be required. This will be quickly confirmed if you go straight to hospital, where the doctor or midwife can observe you very carefully.

Vacuum extraction

The vacuum extractor, or ventouse, is a gentler alternative to forceps, and is widely used throughout Europe. It consists of a metal plate or cup of synthetic material, which is placed over the baby's scalp.

Using an attached pump, a vacuum is created that makes the plate or cup adhere. This instrument then becomes a "handle" with which the obstetrician can both rotate the head and apply traction. Although it leaves a conspicuous bruise to the baby's head, it has many advantages:

✳ The device takes up less room in the vagina and is easier to apply than forceps.

✳ It can be applied before the cervix is fully dilated and with less discomfort than forceps.

✳ It can be applied to the lowest part of the baby's head.

✳ The shape of the baby's head is unaffected.

✳ An episiotomy is not usually necessary.

Special deliveries

The usual course of delivery is set out in the previous pages. Certain factors, however, may complicate a delivery and special procedures may be required. Sometimes a delivery is different because the complicating factor may not have been anticipated, and forceps or a vacuum extractor will have to be used. On the other hand, multiple and breech births are special but are usually diagnosed well in advance.

Assisted delivery

Occasionally, labour and delivery do not proceed as smoothly as expected, so your obstetrician will require assistance to complete a vaginal delivery. Forceps (see p. 75) can be used to protect the baby's head, or may be used, along with vacuum extraction (see column, left), to accelerate the baby's progress through the birth canal.

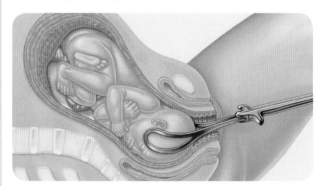

Forceps extraction In a forceps delivery, your baby's head is cradled on either side with metal tongs that guide him down the birth canal – without too much compression – in time with your contractions.

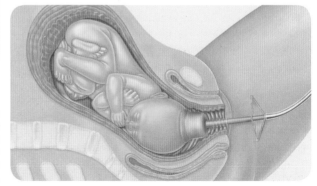

Ventouse extraction With ventouse assistance, a small suction plate or cup is attached by vacuum to the lowest part of the baby's head. The doctor will gradually help the baby to be born by applying gentle traction.

Multiple deliveries

The delivery of twins is always approached as if there were two single babies, because if one has a vaginal delivery it does not follow that the other one will too. Almost certainly, you will be advised to have the babies in hospital in case they are not lying properly. However, the most common way for twin babies to lie at birth is for them both to be head down. The second one usually arrives 8–10 minutes after the first. Your obstetrician will probably recommend an epidural anaesthetic (see p. 43), as twin labours can be prolonged, or the second baby may have to be turned. This is done by rupturing the second baby's membrane and manually moving the baby into the correct position.

Twin deliveries have become much safer in recent years because the exact position and condition of the second baby can be confirmed by ultrasound scanning and fetal monitoring. If you are expecting three or more babies, it is more likely that you will have a Caesarean section, although some doctors will deliver triplets vaginally if they have great experience in this procedure.

Breech birth

If your baby is in a breech position (buttocks down), and you and your obstetrician decide that he can be delivered safely without a Caesarean section, he will be born vaginally. The breech birth should not be thought of as an abnormal birth – it is better to think of it as a variation of normal, because 4 out of every 100 babies are born in the breech position and most of them arrive smoothly, and are healthy.

In most breech births, the buttocks are delivered first, then the legs. The body slips out next. Before the head is delivered, you will almost certainly have to have an episiotomy because the head is the widest part and your baby's bottom will not have stretched your birth canal sufficiently for his head to pass through it without some pressure being applied.

Once the baby's body is born, his weight pulls the head down. His body is then lifted upwards by the midwife, and one more push is usually enough to deliver him. Forceps may be used to protect the baby's head (see column, right).

It is now fairly common practice for you to be given an epidural if you are having a breech birth. This is so that if you need a Caesarean section it can be done quickly and simply without further anaesthesia, and you will be able to hold your baby as soon as he is born.

Forceps delivery

Forceps look like large sugar tongs and are designed so that they will fit snugly over the sides of the baby's head, covering the ears. They're rather like a cage and protect the head from any pressure within the birth canal.

The decision to use forceps is a medical one. Forceps are only applied when the first stage is complete, the cervix is fully dilated, and the head is in the birth canal.

Why it is done Forceps are used when the baby's head has descended into the mother's pelvis but fails to descend further; when the baby is presenting in a posterior position or in a breech delivery (see left); when the uterus fails to maintain contractions; or when the mother lacks the strength to push out her baby.

How it is done You will be asked to lie on your back and your legs will be put up in stirrups. A local anaesthetic will be injected into your perineum, and an episiotomy performed. Then the forceps will be inserted into your vagina one at a time. A few gentle pulls on the forceps, 30–40 seconds at a time, will bring your baby's head out. The rest of his body will be delivered as usual.

On your way to the hospital

If the urge to bear down comes as you are driving to the hospital, use your breathing techniques to avoid pushing; try to remain calm.

Assess the situation with your partner. If the urge is too strong for you to control, your partner should pull the car over and stop. If possible, cover the back seat and car floor with a thick layer of newspapers or towels. You can then lie down on the back seat and deliver the baby into your partner's hands.

If you are the carer, you should follow the procedure for the birth (see right). If the placenta arrives before you reach hospital, wrap it up with the baby, because this provides him with much needed extra warmth. Place blankets or towels over your partner (who may well be shivering by this time), so that she and the baby are well covered, especially the baby's head, as most of the heat is lost from here. Bear in mind that the normal colour of a baby at birth is bluish-white. He will gradually become pink in the first minutes as oxygen enters his body; his hands and feet will take somewhat longer.

Sudden birth

Sometimes labour progresses so quickly that the birth happens away from medical assistance, whether at home or on the way to hospital. If this happens, the following information will help you and your partner deliver your baby safely.

This is not intended to be used as a guide for an out-of-hospital birth without a professional attendant being present, as this can be very risky indeed. Be reassured that the majority of emergency births that happen at home do not suffer any complications.

What you should do

As you get the urge to push, try to pant or blow for as long as you can in order to delay your baby's birth. However, the contractions alone are usually enough to expel the baby when he is coming this fast, so this will not delay things for long, although it may be long enough for your midwife or the ambulance to arrive. Never try to hold your legs together to delay delivery, or allow anyone else to do so, as it may result in your baby having brain damage.

If you cannot comfortably delay your baby's birth, don't try to interfere. Deliver the head slowly. There is a greater chance that your vagina and perineum will tear if you push along with the force of your uterus, so pant lightly with each contraction.

Prolapsed cord If a loop of the umbilical cord washes out when the membranes rupture and your partner can see a piece of grey-blue shiny cord bulging out of your vagina, this means that you have a prolapsed cord and you must get help as soon as possible because your baby's oxygen supply is in danger of being cut off. Don't panic; there is time. Get on to the floor on your knees, with your chest to your knees, your head on the floor, and raise your buttocks in the air. This will help to take the pressure of the baby's head off your cervix.

If the cord is still protruding, your partner should cover it with a wet, warm, very clean towel while he rings the hospital or goes for help. Do not touch or put any pressure on the cord and stay in the knee-chest position even on the way to hospital, because it reduces pressure on the cord. A prolapsed cord nearly always necessitates a Caesarean delivery.

What the birth assistant should do

If it looks as though the baby will be born at home without medical assistance, you should telephone the hospital or the midwife if you haven't done so already. If you haven't got a telephone, on no account should you leave the mother alone. However anxious and overwhelmed you are, you must stay calm and reassure her – she needs to feel confident and relaxed. Encourage her to take up any position in which she feels comfortable (see pp. 48–49), and to eat and drink if she feels like it. Speak quietly and keep any onlookers at bay.

Between contractions Turn up the heating in the room if at all possible. Wash your hands thoroughly with soap and water, and then fetch several clean bath towels and place them conveniently at hand. Fold one and put it on the bed or the floor so that you have something soft on which the baby can be laid.

Then fill several bowls with hand-warm water and collect as many clean hand towels, face flannels, or tea-towels as you can; immerse these in the water to use as wipes for the mother and baby during and after delivery.

The birth Your partner will know when the baby is coming because she'll feel a stinging or burning sensation as the baby stretches her vagina. After washing your hands thoroughly again, look to see if you can see the top of the baby's head in the vaginal outlet (known as crowning – see pp. 53 and 55). Remind your partner to pant or blow, so that her vagina and perineum have time to thin and stretch, which may help her to avoid tearing.

The baby's head will probably be born in one contraction and the rest of his body in the contraction afterwards. When the head is born, wipe each of the baby's eyes from inside to outside with separate pieces of moist linen, and then feel his neck to see if the cord is wrapped around it. If it is, crook your little finger underneath it and pull it very gently over the head, or lift it so that the body can be born through the loop.

Do not cut the cord, because it may go into a spasm and deprive your baby of oxygen. If the membranes (called the caul) are still present over the baby's face, gently tear them off so that the baby can breathe. Hold the baby firmly, as he will be slippery with blood, mucus, and a waxy substance called *vernix caseosa*. Be careful not to pull on his head, his body, or the cord.

Delivery of the placenta

Keep these points in mind if the placenta is delivered before an attendant arrives:

* Never cut or pull on the cord.

* After the placenta comes out, massage the mother's abdomen firmly, with a deep circular motion, gently pushing downwards 5–7cm (2–3in) below the navel. This is important to make sure the uterus contracts and stays hard after the birth to prevent haemorrhaging.

* It's normal for a couple of cups of blood to be delivered when the placenta comes out.

* Encourage the mother to nurse her baby immediately, as this will help contract the uterus and minimize blood loss.

After the birth

Once the baby is born, he will probably give a couple of gasps, a cry, and then start to cry properly.

If he doesn't cry, place him across your partner's thigh or abdomen, with his head lower than his feet, and then gently rub his back. This helps any mucus drain away and usually causes a change in blood pressure, which will bring about his first breath.

Incision

The Caesarean incision It is now more usual to have a short horizontal cut rather than a vertical one because a horizontal cut is believed to heal faster. It is usually made below the shaved pubic ("bikini") hairline.

Caesarean section

When a normal vaginal delivery is considered dangerous or even impossible, your baby will be delivered by Caesarean section – an operation where horizontal incisions are made in your abdomen and uterus, and your baby is delivered through them. (The old-fashioned vertical cut is not used nowadays because it is more likely to tear during a subsequent labour.) The percentage of babies delivered by Caesarean section has increased rapidly, and is currently around 18–20 per cent in the United Kingdom, and over 20 per cent in the United States. This is partly because doctors are worried about being sued if a difficult birth causes complications that could have been avoided by Caesarean section, and partly because the operation is now so safe that it can be less risky than some other kinds of delivery.

What happens

Very often, when a Caesarean section is necessary, the need for it will be apparent before labour begins, which means that you, your partner, and the obstetrician have time to discuss and plan for it. This type of planned Caesarean, known as elective, is in contrast to an emergency Caesarean, where the need for it may only become evident once labour is underway.

Preparation You are given the spinal or epidural anaesthetic (see p. 43), and an intravenous drip is set up to supply you with fluids during the operation. Then a catheter (a thin, flexible tube) is inserted up your urethra and into your bladder to drain it of urine. Before the operation begins, your pubic hair is shaved and your abdomen is swabbed with antiseptic. This kills off any bacteria on the skin that could enter your body via the incision. A small screen is placed in front of your face so that you and your partner can't see the operation.

The operation The obstetrician makes a short, horizontal incision along the "bikini line" at the base of your abdomen, then makes a similar incision in the lower segment of your uterus. The amniotic fluid is drained off by suction, and the baby is gently lifted out. Then the cord is cut, the placenta is removed, and your uterus and abdomen are stitched. A Caesarean operation usually takes 45–60 minutes, but the baby is delivered within the first 5–10 minutes; the rest is spent stitching you.

Elective Caesarean section

The most common reasons for deciding to have a Caesarean include the baby being in a breech position (see p. 75) or lying across your pelvis; the baby's head being too large to pass through your pelvis; placenta praevia (where the placenta has implanted near or over the cervix); and certain medical conditions such as diabetes.

It may also be necessary if you have previously had a Caesarean. This was once thought essential, because it was feared that the scar of the previous Caesarean section would open up during labour. But experience has shown that this does not happen with the horizontal or "bikini" cut, which is now usually employed. Doctors often suggest that you try a normal vaginal delivery, known as a VBAC (vaginal birth after Caesarean). However, remember that it is your uterus that is on trial, not you, so don't feel you have failed if you end up having another Caesarean.

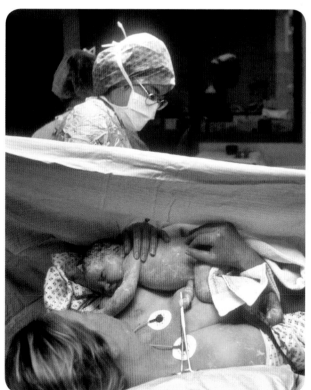

Caesarean with an epidural
Caesareans are now rarely performed under a full anaesthetic, but you are given an epidural or spinal anaesthetic, which numbs the lower part of your body. It also means that you can be conscious throughout the operation and your partner can be with you. The procedure is very quick – within 5–10 minutes of the incisions being made the baby is delivered and you are able to hold your new son or daughter.

The effects on your baby

Not having to pass through the birth canal is both a benefit and a drawback for the baby born by Caesarean section.

Unlike a baby born by vaginal delivery, who initially has a rather squashed appearance after being squeezed through the birth canal, a Caesarean baby has smooth features and a rounded head. But often, the Caesarean baby needs more time to adjust to the outside world because of his sudden entry into it, and because he has missed the journey through the birth canal that helps to clear amniotic fluid from a baby's lungs and stimulates his circulation.

The use of spinal or epidural anaesthesia has several advantages over a general anaesthetic: it is safer for your baby, you have no post-operative nausea or vomiting, and because you are conscious, you can hold your baby as soon as he is born. In addition, it is usually possible for your partner to be with you during the operation, just as he would be if you were having a vaginal delivery.

When you have a Caesarean, you may feel disappointed or even cheated that you did not have a vaginal delivery. Such feelings are perfectly natural, and the best thing you can do is talk about them with your partner. It will probably help if he describes the birth to you in detail – this will help you to visualize and accept it better.

It also helps, of course, to prepare yourself in advance for this type of birth. With your partner present, find out from the obstetrician what the operation entails, what procedures will be used, and whether your partner will be allowed to be present. Ask if you can see a video of the operation, so that you know what is going to happen to you. If at all possible, talk to other women who have had Caesarean sections. They will not only provide you with useful information but also with emotional and moral support.

Emergency Caesarean section

This is often needed when something goes wrong during labour, such as a prolapsed umbilical cord or haemorrhage from the placenta, or if there is evidence of fetal distress. Most commonly, it is performed for prolonged labour, where a vaginal delivery is thought to be unlikely.

After a Caesarean section

As is the case with any major surgery, it takes time to recover from a Caesarean, but even so you will be encouraged to get up and walk around a few hours afterwards to stimulate your circulation. You'll be given painkillers if you need them, and the dressings will be removed after three or four days. Your internal stitches are made with absorbable sutures, which will dissolve away naturally, and your external stitches will be removed within about a week.

Chapter 6

Getting back to normal

Plan to **take some time off** just after the birth. Give yourself **time and space** to get to know and **bond with your new baby**. Don't feel you have to get back to normal immediately.

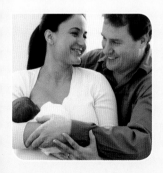

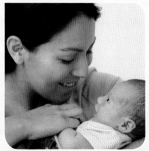

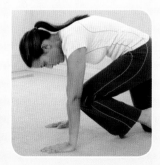

Postnatal changes

The sudden change in hormone levels following childbirth is thought to be a principal cause of the so-called "baby blues" and postnatal depression.

Very soon after you conceive, the levels of certain hormones in your body, especially progesterone and oestrogen, rise steeply and stay elevated throughout the months of pregnancy. Then, during the first 72 hours after giving birth, the levels of these hormones crash.

When the levels of oestrogen and progesterone drop so suddenly and drastically, your body finds it difficult to adjust. This can have a marked effect on your emotions and mental processes, and with other factors, such as relationship problems, may lead to baby blues or even postnatal depression.

Severe exhaustion, another possible problem, can be made worse by a lack of potassium in your body. This is easily corrected by eating plenty of potassium-rich foods, such as bananas or tomatoes.

Your changing emotions

During the days and weeks following the birth, you will be in an emotionally fluctuating state because of the abrupt reduction in your pregnancy hormones (see column, left). And, because it is such a major event in your life, giving birth is liable to accentuate any underlying personal or emotional problems you may have, and to resurrect any unresolved issues. It is therefore difficult to predict just how you will react to the birth of your baby – sometimes an elated, trouble-free pregnancy can be followed by a low-key postnatal period. The nature, severity, and duration of postnatal problems can vary greatly from one woman to another, and from one pregnancy to another. A woman can have a trouble-free postnatal period after one pregnancy, then have a rough time following a subsequent birth.

The "baby blues"

Because the most important single cause of postnatal emotional problems is the abrupt and unavoidable drop in hormone levels, you should not be surprised if, like most women after giving birth, you suffer from the baby blues to some extent. As many as 80 per cent of mothers do, so it really is the norm rather than the exception, and women who escape it entirely are in a fortunate minority. For the nine months of pregnancy, you have been experiencing very high levels of hormones and suddenly you are plunged back to the comparatively low levels of normality. This drastic but normal swing renders the majority of women weepy, prone to sudden mood swings, irritable, indecisive, and anxious.

The baby blues usually set in about three to five days after the birth and last for about a week to 10 days. The onset often coincides with the beginning of your milk production (which itself is governed by your changing hormones) and for this reason the baby blues were known in the 19th century as "milk fever".

Becoming a mother If you do get the baby blues, you usually find that the reality of being a mother seems quite difficult to cope with once the initial euphoria of having your new baby in your arms wears off. In addition to the symptoms mentioned above, you might find yourself confused, anxious about your ability to look after your baby, and frustrated because it seems to be taking you so long to learn to be a good mother. Be easy on yourself; no woman has the expertise for instant motherhood – this is something that can be acquired only through learning, which takes time.

It is also important not to overdo things. Tiredness is inevitable in the early days, but it should never be ignored. If you feel tired, stop whatever you are doing if it's not essential, and lie down with your feet raised slightly above your head. You don't have to go to sleep to conserve your strength; a good rest may be all you need.

Postnatal depression

About 10 per cent of all mothers develop postnatal depression (PND). This is, in many respects, quite different and separate from the baby blues. PND is longer-lasting, more serious, and needs immediate medical attention. It is a psychiatric disorder that can get out of hand if left untreated, and it is absolutely essential that you seek medical help early. With treatment, your depression will normally resolve itself in a few weeks; the longer PND is left untreated, the longer it will take to resolve.

Symptoms There are many symptoms associated with PND, and these are experienced by different women in different combinations. In addition to depressive symptoms, such as hopelessness and despondency, sufferers can experience lethargy, anxiety, tension, panic, sleep difficulties, loss of interest in sex, obsessional thoughts, feelings of guilt, and a lack of self-esteem.

Treatment Drugs will help you recover from postnatal depression, but support from family and friends is also vital. There are also some things you can do for yourself (see column, right). Your doctor will normally prescribe antidepressant drugs. Over a period of time, these will bring about a gentle and gradual improvement, so it's important to keep taking your medication even after you start feeling better. Some drugs may have minor side-effects, such as drowsiness or confused thoughts. Don't be afraid to ask your doctor for alternative treatments if you are concerned.

If you find that your feelings of depression get worse just before your period, tell your doctor. He or she may be able to prescribe further medication, to prevent this severe form of premenstrual syndrome.

Self-help for depression

If you are feeling low, there are a number of things you can do to help yourself. The most important thing is to believe that you will get better, no matter how much time it takes.

Rest as much as possible Tiredness makes depression worse and harder to cope with. Catnap during the day and try getting help with night feeds.

Maintain a proper diet Eat plenty of fruit or raw vegetables – don't snack or binge on chocolates and sweet biscuits. Eat little and often. Do not go on a strict diet.

Take gentle exercise Give yourself a break from being indoors or taking care of the baby. A brisk walk in the fresh air can help lift your spirits.

Avoid major upheavals Don't move house or redecorate.

Try not to worry unduly Aches and pains are common after childbirth, and more so if you are depressed. They will probably ease as you relax.

Be kind to yourself Don't force yourself to do things you don't want to or that might upset you. Don't worry about keeping the house spotless.

Talk about it Bottling up your concerns will make it worse. Talk to your partner or friends.

What is lochia?

While your uterus contracts and returns to its normal condition and size after delivery, you will have a vaginal discharge known as lochia.

Lochia is the normal vaginal discharge from a healing uterus. The duration of lochia loss varies widely from woman to woman. Its average length is about 21 days, although it may be as short as 14 days or continue for up to six weeks. Breastfeeding may help to reduce the duration of lochia, because the hormone that triggers the breastmilk also causes uterine contractions, which help reduce bleeding.

However long it continues, lochia flow goes through three distinct stages. For the first three or four days, the lochia is bright red, then it gradually reduces in quantity and changes to pink or brown, eventually becoming yellowish-white or colourless.

Lochia should have a fresh, blood-like odour; if it becomes at all foul-smelling, consult your doctor at once because this may indicate an infection. Also tell your doctor if the flow suddenly becomes bright red again. This usually means that the uterus is not healing well, perhaps due to over-exertion.

Because there is a risk of infection, you should not use tampons until about six weeks after delivery, so use sanitary towels until the lochia ceases.

Your postnatal health

After childbirth, your body begins to reverse the changes that it went through during pregnancy and labour. The withdrawal of the huge amounts of pregnancy hormones is like the withdrawal of a life force, and this period – known as the postnatal or postpartum period – can be a very tiring one for you. Try to get as much rest and relaxation as you can, and also make sure that your diet is healthy, and includes an adequate amount of fluids (at least a pint of milk a day and four pints of other liquids). If you are breastfeeding, you will need to take good care of your breasts and nipples (see p. 86).

Pelvic area

After delivery, your uterus, cervix, vagina, and abdomen begin to shrink back to approximately their pre-pregnant size and pre-labour state. The shrinkage of your uterus is accompanied by a vaginal discharge known as lochia (see column, left) and by contractions or cramps called afterpains.

Afterpains All women feel uterine contractions throughout their fertile lives. During menstruation, they are known as menstrual cramps, during pregnancy as Braxton Hicks' contractions, and following delivery as afterpains. After delivery, uterine contractions are the means by which the uterus returns to its former non-pregnant size; the faster and harder it contracts the better. You may also feel these pains when you breastfeed, because the hormone oxytocin involved in milk production also causes uterine contractions.

Bowels and bladder You should get out of bed to use the toilet as soon as you possibly can after delivery. However, if you emptied your bowels before or during the delivery, you may not feel the need for 24 hours or more, and this is quite normal. When you have a bowel movement you may feel the urge to bear down. Any pressure in the perineal region will stretch your tissues and cause pain if you have an episiotomy wound (see p. 85). To prevent this, hold a clean pad firmly against the stitches and press upwards while you bear down. Do everything you can to prevent constipation and the need to strain. Eat lots of fibre, especially vegetables and fruit, and drink plenty of water (see p. 87). Drinking plenty of water, in addition to getting up and walking about, will help get both your bowels and your bladder working normally. There may be some hesitation before the urine starts to flow for the first time. This is nothing to worry about, and is usually the result of the swelling of the perineum and tissues around the urethral opening. Urine flow can be triggered by the sound of running water, so try turning on the bathroom taps while you sit on the lavatory.

Cervix and vagina These will have been stretched considerably and will be soft and slack for a while. It takes about a week for your cervix to narrow and firm up again, which it will do unaided, but you can speed up the recovery of your vagina by contracting and relaxing its muscles, by doing pelvic floor exercises (see p. 11). You should begin these exercises within about 24 hours of giving birth. You can also use exercises to tone up your abdominal muscles (see pp. 88–89), but do not begin these until the flow of lochia has stopped.

Caesarean wound If you have had a Caesarean section, you should avoid abdominal exercises and lifting heavy weights for the first six weeks or until the wound has completely healed. Try not to climb stairs more than once a day, be careful how you move when getting up from a lying or sitting position, and generally try not to put any strain on your abdominal muscles.

Haemorrhoids Also known as piles, these are quite common after childbirth; they are caused by the great strain imposed on the veins in the pelvic floor during labour and delivery. They appear as lumpy swellings just inside your anus, and with proper care (consult your doctor or midwife) they will eventually shrink away.

Menstruation and ovulation

Menstruation and ovulation will resume some time between eight and 16 weeks after delivery, but both may be significantly delayed if you are breastfeeding. However, if you want to resume making love before your periods have started, you must use birth control because ovulation will precede menstruation.

Breasts and nipples

The increased size and weight of your breasts will mean that you need a good quality, well-fitting cotton maternity bra both for convenience and comfort. Wear a clean one every day, and

The episiotomy wound

The pain from an episiotomy wound gets worse before it gets better. The wound is positioned where fluid can accumulate in the cut edges. These then swell, with the result that the stitches become tighter and bite into the sore skin around the wound.

If you are bruised or if the stitches are really painful, it will help to sit on an inflatable rubber ring (some hospitals have these). Good hygiene is vitally important while the wound is healing, so make sure that it is kept clean. Most stitches will dissolve after five or six days.

Warm baths and showers are soothing and encourage the healing process, as do pelvic-floor exercises. You may also find that ice packs or local anaesthetic creams are helpful. There are special perineal pads available that fit between your sanitary towel and the wound. Your doctor or midwife will advise you about these.

Don't use antiseptics or perfumed bubble liquid in your bath water because they can cause irritation. After bathing, dry the area with a hairdryer instead of a towel, which can be painful.

Urine, which is acidic, will make the raw skin sting. Standing up to urinate may help. Try pouring warm water over yourself as you're urinating, to dilute the acid and reduce the sting.

Combating fatigue

Getting enough rest and sleep is essential if you are to combat the inevitable fatigue of the first weeks of caring for your newborn baby.

Try to rest whenever you can, especially during the first week or so when you will still be recovering from the exhaustion of labour. Avoid climbing stairs and heavy lifting as much as possible, and get your partner or someone else to help you with the baby and the general housework. Take advantage of your baby's daytime naps to rest or nap yourself, and try not to waste these valuable chances for rest by using them to catch up on the ever-present chores.

Make sure that you get enough sleep. At night, go to bed half an hour or so before you plan on going to sleep, and unwind slowly. Try sipping a warm, milky drink, listening to music, watching television, or doing a little light reading to relax you physically and mentally before you sleep.

If you are breastfeeding, express milk into bottles so that your partner can share the night-time feeding duties just as he would if you are bottle-feeding.

A healthy diet is an essential part of combating fatigue, but avoid eating too much late at night as the digesting of food might interfere with your normal sleep pattern.

if you are using breast pads to prevent leaking milk from staining your clothes, avoid those that are backed with plastic. Change the pads after each feed and whenever they become wet.

Care of your breasts Clean your breasts and nipples daily with cotton wool and baby lotion or water, but avoid using soap because it strips away the natural oils that protect the skin from drying and cracking, and it can aggravate a sore or cracked nipple. Always treat your breasts with care – don't rub them dry for example, but very gently pat them dry instead.

There is no need to wash your nipples before or after each feed, but before you fasten or put on your bra after feeding, let your nipples dry in the air, and always wash your hands before handling your breasts in order to prevent infection.

Engorgement About three or four days after you have given birth, your breasts will fill with milk. They will become larger and heavier, and feel tender and warm when you touch them. If they overfill, the condition is known as engorgement. This usually only lasts a day or two, but it can be uncomfortable and may recur.

To ease engorged breasts, take off milk either by expressing manually or by feeding your baby (you may have to express a little milk first so that he can latch on). In addition, you may find that it helps to bathe your breasts with warm water, cover them with warm towels, or to stroke them gently but firmly towards the nipple.

Engorgement can recur at any time while breastfeeding, particularly if your breasts are never properly emptied or if your baby misses a feed.

Blocked ducts A blocked milk duct may occur in the early weeks of breastfeeding. It may result from engorgement, from a bra that is too tight, or from dried secretions on the nipple tip. Your breast will feel tender and lumpy and there may be a reddening of the skin.

To clear a blocked duct, start feeds with the affected breast and gently massage it just above the sore area while feeding, to ease the milk gently towards the nipple. If the blockage does not clear, don't offer that breast to your baby and consult your doctor immediately because it could become infected.

Sore nipples When you begin breastfeeding, your nipples may feel slightly tender or very sore for the first minute or so of suckling. This tenderness is quite normal, and it usually disappears after a few days. Prolonged sore nipples, however, can turn what should be a pleasure into something of an ordeal. Take care when latching on and taking your baby off your breasts, to prevent these problems from arising. This is also essential if the nipples are to heal after they have become sore or cracked.

Cracked nipples If a sore nipple becomes cracked, you may need to keep the baby off that breast for up to 72 hours and express milk from the breast to avoid engorgement. Cracked nipples can be very painful, and they can lead to breast infection (mastitis).

Protecting sore nipples

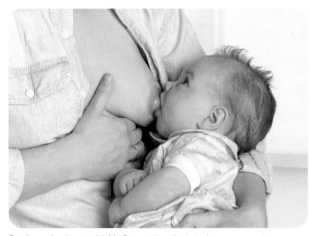

Feeding using breast shields Sore and cracked nipples are a common problem in the early weeks of breastfeeeding. If your nipples get sore, use breast shields to protect them during feeding. Your baby will adjust quickly to the feel and taste of the shield.

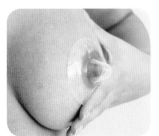

Wearing a breast shield Ease your nipple into the shield by slipping your hand between breast and ribcage and pushing gently upwards. The shield will fit over the nipple and the baby will suck through it.

Dealing with constipation

Many women suffer from constipation after giving birth. If you find you are affected, exercise, a sensible diet, and drinking lots of fluid will help you to deal with it.

After delivery, the passage of faeces through your bowels tends to slow down, and this can lead to constipation. The slowing down occurs mainly because your abdominal muscles are relaxed and stretched and so the pressure within your abdomen is lower than normal. Relaxation of the bowel muscles themselves because of the high levels of progesterone during pregnancy may also slow down bowel movements. If you have had an episiotomy you might, consciously or unconsciously, hold back from passing stools for fear of causing pain.

Medication such as laxatives, stool softeners, or suppositories can help get things moving again, but if you are breastfeeding it is best to avoid taking medication because it can be passed to your baby via your milk, and can cause stomach cramps and watery stools.

The best remedies for constipation (and a good way to prevent it) are to eat prunes or figs, drink plenty of fluids, eat lots of fibre-rich foods, and avoid inactivity by getting out and about if you feel up to it.

Exercises for the first days

You can do a few gentle exercises just days after giving birth. Whether lying in bed or sitting on a chair, try to get into the habit of toning your muscles regularly.

Your pelvic floor muscles are very important and exercising them will strengthen them and prevent incontinence.

Tone up your pelvic floor and stomach muscles by pulling them in as you breathe out, then holding for a few seconds. Relax, and then repeat as often as possible.

You can prevent, or reduce, swollen ankles and feet simply by circling your feet as you sit.

Postnatal exercises

A few weeks after giving birth, try to establish a daily exercise routine. This may not seem like a top priority when you're faced with the new demands of being a mother; however, exercising will tone muscles that were stretched during pregnancy and delivery, and increase your energy supply. It's also good for your morale and will enhance your feeling of wellbeing. Exercise twice or several times a day rather than for one long period.

If you've had a Caesarean, wait for four to six weeks before starting to exercise, and check with your doctor first. If you have had an episiotomy or a tear, don't practise stretching exercises until it has healed.

Forward bend

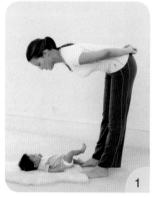 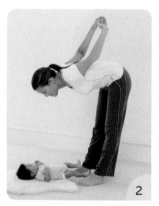

1 Bend forward Place your feet 30cm (12in) apart, keeping them parallel, and loosely clasp your hands behind your back. Keeping your back straight, bend slowly forward from your hips.

2 Raise your arms Then raise your hands until they are as far above your head as you can possibly reach. Breathe deeply for a few breaths, then rise slowly and repeat.

Abdominal toner

Tone your stomach Lie on your back on the floor with your knees bent, your feet flat on the floor, and your arms by your sides. Breathe deeply. As you breathe out, tense your stomach muscles and raise your head and arms, palms downward. Hold for a couple of seconds, then relax. Repeat 10 times. You'll be able to lift your head higher with practice.

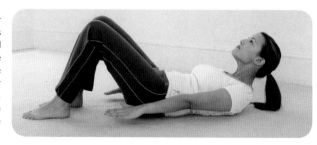

Cat arching

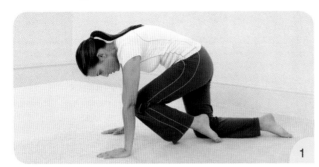

1 Stretch your back Start by kneeling on all fours with your back straight. Breathing in, bend a leg up and lower your forehead towards your knee. Hold for a second.

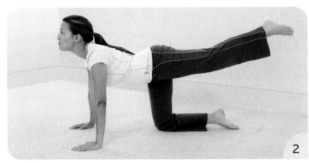

2 Straighten your leg Breathing out, lift your head up, and stretch your neck and push your chin forward, raising the leg behind you. Hold for a few seconds, then change legs.

Side bends

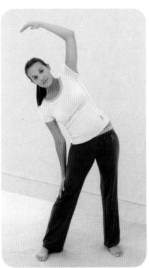

Stretch sideways Stand with your feet about shoulder-width apart. With your right hand on your thigh, slowly bend over to the right. Run your right hand down your leg as far as you can without straining, raise your left hand over your head, and breathe deeply. Try to keep your pelvis level. Hold your breath for a short while, then straighten up as you breathe out. Repeat the exercise, bending over to the other side.

Pelvic tuck-in

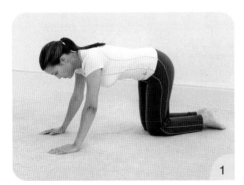

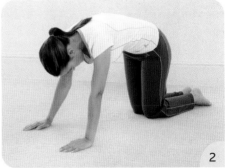

1 Kneel down This exercise helps to correct the tilt of your pelvis. Kneel down on all fours. Keep your back straight and don't let it sag.

2 Arch upwards Tighten your buttock muscles, tuck in your pelvis, and arch your back upwards into a hump. Hold for a few seconds, and release. Repeat several times.

Considering sex

You probably won't be in the mood for making love in the first days, or even weeks, after giving birth, because the sheer physical exhaustion of labour and the drastic changes in your hormone levels after delivery combine to inhibit sexual desire. An initial lack of interest in sex is both natural and desirable, because your body needs time to recover from the changes and stress of pregnancy and childbirth, and you need time to adjust to your new baby. Talk to your partner – he will probably be sympathetic and understanding.

Your partner

The arrival of the baby can also have a dampening effect on your partner's libido; it is not uncommon for a father to feel a temporary lack of desire and even to lose his ability to maintain an erection, and he might find it difficult to adjust to his and your dual, sometimes contradictory, roles as lovers and parents.

Both of you must be prepared for such problems and should not take them personally. If you are philosophical and open about your problems, and discuss them lovingly and sympathetically with each other, you will prevent them from developing into long-term difficulties.

When to give it a go

The point at which sexual desire returns varies greatly from one couple to another, and even from one pregnancy to another. There is also the question of just when it is physically safe for intercourse; couples were once advised to give up sex six weeks before the expected date of delivery and to abstain from it for six weeks afterwards (until after the six-week check). This well-meaning advice is now thought to be unnecessarily cautious, and the general opinion today is that penetrative sex can continue as late in pregnancy as you wish – provided there are no medical reasons to avoid it – and that you can begin again when you feel up to it. You can also have non-penetrative sex before and after giving birth whenever you feel like it.

If both of you are feeling happy about it, and there is no medical objection, you can resume sexual activity as soon as you feel the desire. In addition, making love can have a beneficial effect for a number of reasons. For example, it reaffirms your affection and desire for each other, and the hormones released during sexual activity cause contractions of your uterus, which will help it return to its pre-pregnant state.

Lack of desire

Don't worry about loss of libido – it's natural. There are many factors that can conspire against your desire for and enjoyment of postnatal sex. Apart from any lingering discomfort you might feel, it is quite common for women to see themselves as unattractive at first, and this can make them shy away from sex or think negatively. Your still-bulging tummy may make you feel unsexy, so starting exercises to get back into shape is important for your self-esteem (see pp. 88–89). Remember that doing pelvic floor exercises will help reduce the slackness of your vagina.

Anxieties and distractions may also diminish your sexual desire or enjoyment. Fear of getting pregnant again may bother you, and resuming birth control can be worrying or annoying. Even your baby can have a considerable influence on your enjoyment of lovemaking, because you may not feel as free as before, or as able to abandon yourself while you half-expect your baby to cry for attention at any time.

It is also possible for you to get so absorbed with your baby that you find you have little need for other emotional ties or physical contact, to the exclusion of your partner. This is because oxytocin, the hormone that is produced during breastfeeding, mimics sexual satisfaction.

Making sex more enjoyable

You might find that it takes a long time for you both to regain your previous level of sexual enjoyment. Both of you need extra fondling, kissing, and other foreplay before you become sexually aroused. For the first few times, you should perhaps avoid penile penetration and stick to gentle oral or manual sex. And because an episiotomy site can be surprisingly painful during intercourse and may take months to become pain-free, be honest with your partner and tell him if sex causes you discomfort or pain. Getting him to feel your scar may help him to understand. A warm bath before lovemaking and possibly a vaginal lubricant or saliva are also a great help. While making love, experiment with other positions – side-by-side positions are good if you're suffering from a sore episiotomy site. Whatever positions you try, be patient, and build up your sexual activity again gradually.

Postnatal check-ups

At about six weeks after delivery, you will visit your GP to be examined.

Your check-up At your visit, you will be weighed and your blood pressure will be checked. You may have a pelvic examination to check that, among other things, your episiotomy has healed well, your cervix has closed, and your uterus is back to normal.

The doctor will usually ask you how you are feeling emotionally, and how you are coping. She or he will also discuss future methods of contraception with you and provide you with a diaphragm (cap) or an IUD should you need one. Even if you used a diaphragm (cap) before, you will now need to be fitted with a new one.

Your baby's six-week check The GP looks at his ears, eyes, limbs, and muscle tone, listens to his heartbeat, checks his control over his head movements, measures the circumference of his head, checks for hip displacements, and weighs him. His weight is recorded on his personal chart at each visit, and is an important record of his progress.

Useful addresses

Active Birth Centre
25 Bickerton Road
London N19 5JT
Tel: 020 7281 6760
www.activebirthcentre.com
*Information and classes on active
involvement in childbirth at home
or in hospital*

Acumedic
101–105 Camden High Street
London NWI 7JN
Tel: 020 7388 6704
www.acumedic.com
*For the hire of a TENS (Transcutaneous
Electrical Nerve Stimulation) machine*

AIMS (Association
for Improvements in
Maternity Services)
5 Ann's Court
Grove Road, Surbiton
Surrey KT6 4BE
Tel: 020 300 365 0663
www.aims.org.uk
*Pressure group that campaigns
for the right of parents to have
the maternity services they want*

APEC (Action on Pre-eclampsia)
2c The Halfcroft
Syston LE7 1LD
Tel: 020 8427 4217
www.apec.org.uk

Aqua Birth Pools
Active Birth Centre
25 Bickerton Road
London N19 5JT
Tel: 020 7281 6760
For the hire of a portable water birth pool

Association of
Breastfeeding Mothers
PO Box 207, Bridgwater
TA6 7YT
Tel: 0844 4122 949
www.abm.me.uk
*A 24-hour telephone service for mothers,
with a network of breastfeeding counsellors*

Association for Postnatal Illness
145 Dawes Road, Fulham
London SW6 7EB
Tel: 020 7386 0868
Advice on coping with postnatal depression

Birthworks
58 Malpas Road
Brockley
London SE4 1BS
Tel: 0333 240 9710
www.birthworks.co.uk
*Advice and literature on water
births; birth pools for hire*

BLISS (Baby Life
Support Systems)
9 Holyrood Street
London SE1 2EL
Tel: 0500 618140
www.bliss.org.uk
*Advice and support for parents
with special-care babies*

British Acupuncture Council
63 Jeddo Road
London W12 9HQ
Tel: 020 8735 0400
www.acupuncture.org.uk

British Epilepsy Association
New Anstey House
Gate Way Drive
Yeadon, Leeds LS19 7XY
Tel: 01132 108800
www.epilepsy.org.uk

British Homeopathic Association
Hahnemann House
29 Park Street West
Luton LU1 3BE
Tel: 01582 408675
www.britishhomeopathic.org

Caesarean Support Network
55 Cooil Drive, Douglas
Isle of Man IM2 2HF
Tel: 01624 661269 (after 6 pm)

Chelsea and
Westminster Hospital
369 Fulham Road
London SW10 9NH
Tel: 020 8746 8000
www.chelwest.nhs.uk
Contact for birth plan information

CHILD
Charter House
43 St. Leonard's Road
Bexhill-on-Sea,
East Sussex TN40 1JA

Tel: 0800 008 7464
www.infertilitynetworkuk.com
*Advice and support for
couples experiencing infertility*

Diabetes UK (formerly the
British Diabetic Association)
Macleod House, 10 Parkway
London NW1 7AA
Tel: 020 7424 1000
www.diabetes.org.uk
Advice for pregnant women with diabetes

Down's Syndrome Association
Langdon Down Centre, 2a Langdon
Park, Teddington TW11 9PS
Tel: 0845 230 0372
www.downs-syndrome.org.uk
*Advice on the care of children
with Down's syndrome*

Freeline Social Security Number
0800 882200
*Free helpline for information about
maternity benefits*

Gingerbread
255 Kentish Town Road
London NW5 2LX
Tel: 0808 802 0925
www.gingerbread.org.uk
*A mutual support group for
one-parent families*

Independent Midwives'
Association
PO box 539
Abingdon OX14 9DF
Tel: 0845 4600 105
www.independentmidwives.org.uk
*Network of independent
midwives offering private care*

La Leche League
129a Middleton Boulevard
Wollaton Park
Nottingham NG8 1FW
Tel: 0845 456 1844
www.laleche.org.uk
*Advice and information
about breastfeeding*

MAMA
54 Lillington Road
Radstock BA3 3NR
Tel: 0845 120 3746

www.mama.co.uk
*Help for new parents, especially
mothers with postnatal depression*

Maternity Action
Tindlemanor, 52-53 Featherstone
Street, London EC1Y 8RT
Tel: 020 7253 2288
www.maternityaction.org.uk
*Information on maternity
rights and benefits*

Miscarriage Association
c/o Clayton Hospital, Northgate
Wakefield
West Yorkshire WF1 3JS
Tel: 01924 200 799
www.miscarriageassociation.org.uk
*Information on a network
of miscarriage support groups*

MS Therapy Centres
7 Peartree Business Centre
Peartree Road, Stanway
Colchester, Essex CO3 0JN
Tel: 0800 783 0518
www.msrc.co.uk
*Information for pregnant
women suffering from MS*

National Childbirth Trust
Alexandra House
Oldham Terrace
London W3 6NH
Tel: 0870 770 3236
www.nctpregnancyandbabycare.com
*Nationwide antenatal classes
and practical postnatal help*

National Childminding Association
Royal Court
81 Tweedy Road, Bromley
Kent BR1 1TG
Tel: 0845 880 0044
www.ncma.org.uk

RCOG (Royal College of Obstetricians and Gynaecologists)
27 Sussex Place
Regent's Park
London NW1 4RG
Tel: 020 7772 6200
www.rcog.org.uk
Helpline and leaflets

Royal College of Midwives
15 Mansfield Street
London W1G 9NH
www.rcm.org.uk
Tel: 020 7312 3535

St Mary's Hospital Recurrent Miscarriage Clinic
Winston Churchill Wing
Praed Street
London W2 1NY
Tel: 020 7886 7777

SANDS (Stillbirth and Neonatal Death Society)
28 Portland Place
London W1B 1LY
Tel: 020 7436 5881
www.uk-sands.org
*National support network
for bereaved parents*

TAMBA (Twins and Multiple Birth Association)
2 The Willows
Gardner Road, Guildford
Surrey GU1 4PG
Tel: 0800 138 0509
www.tamba.org.uk
*Offers encouragement and support for
parents before and after multiple births*

Vegetarian Society
Parkdale Dunham Road
Altrincham
Cheshire WA14 4QG
Tel: 0161 925 2000
www.vegsoc.org
*Nutritional advice for pregnant
women who are vegetarians*

Women's Health
52 Featherstone Street
London EC1Y 8RT
Tel: 020 7251 6580
Advice on reproductive health

Index

Acknowledgments

The publisher would like to thank the following for their kind permission to reproduce their photographs:

(Key: a-above; b-below/bottom; c-centre; f-far; l-left; r-right; t-top)

6 Getty Images: Paul Bradbury. 7 Getty Images: Hans Neleman (bc). 14 Mother & Baby Picture Library: Moose Azim. 17 Alamy Images: Sally and Richard Greenhill. 27 Corbis: Tomas Rodriguez (bc). 34 Corbis: Ragnar Schmuck / fstop (cla). 41 Corbis. 55 Sally & Richard Greenhill (b). 58 Alamy Images: Sally and Richard Greenhill. 61 Alamy Images: Medical-on-Line (bl). Eye Ubiquitous / Hutchison: Nancy Durrell McKenna (fbl) (fbr). Science Photo Library: Ron Sutherland

(cb). 63 Mother & Baby Picture Library: Eddie Lawrence (br). 79 Alamy Images: Janine Wiedel Photolibrary

Jacket images: Front: Mother & Baby Picture Library: Ian Hooton. Back: Getty Images: Ed Fox

DK would like to thank
UK medical consultant: Dr Elizabeth Owen
Proofreader: Angela Baynham

All other images © Dorling Kindersley
For further information see:
www.dkimages.com